The Easy 5-Ingredient
Acid Reflux Cookbook

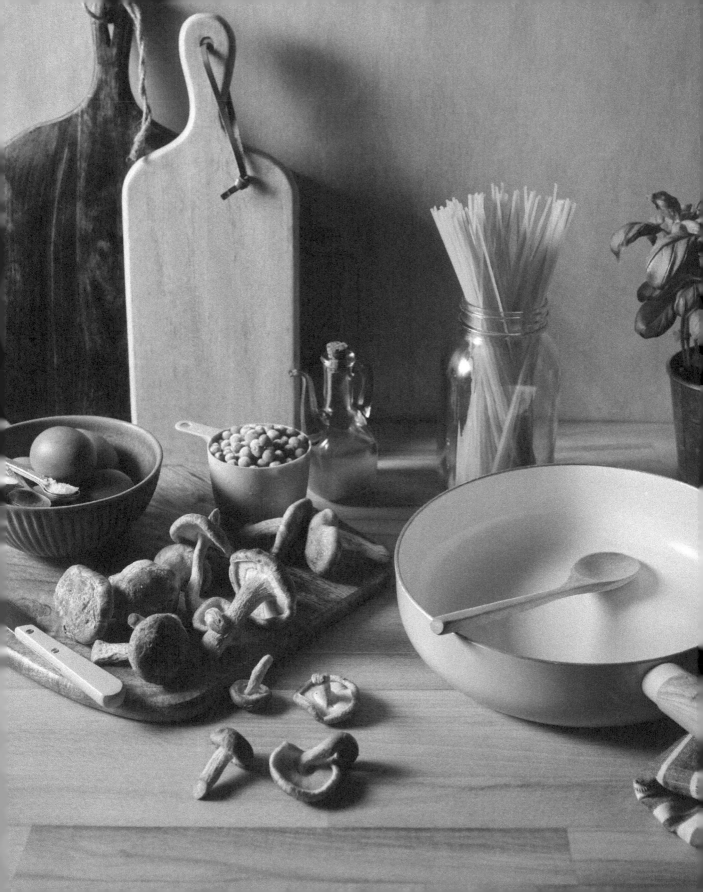

The Easy 5-Ingredient
Acid Reflux
Cookbook

Fuss-Free Recipes
for Relief from GERD and LPR

ANDY DE SANTIS, RD, MPH

Photography by Darren Muir

ROCKRIDGE
PRESS

Interior and Cover Designer: Peatra Jariya
Art Producer: Sue Bischofberger
Editor: Greg Morabito
Production Editor: Emily Sheehan

Photography © 2020 Darren Muir. Author photo courtesy of Natalie CD Photography.

ISBN: Print 978-1-64739-510-0 | eBook 978-1-64739-511-7

R0

◆

This publication is dedicated
to my sister Diana, sometimes
referred to as Dr. De Santis.
I may be the older brother, but your
hard work and accomplishments
inspire and motivate me.
I'm very proud of you!

◆

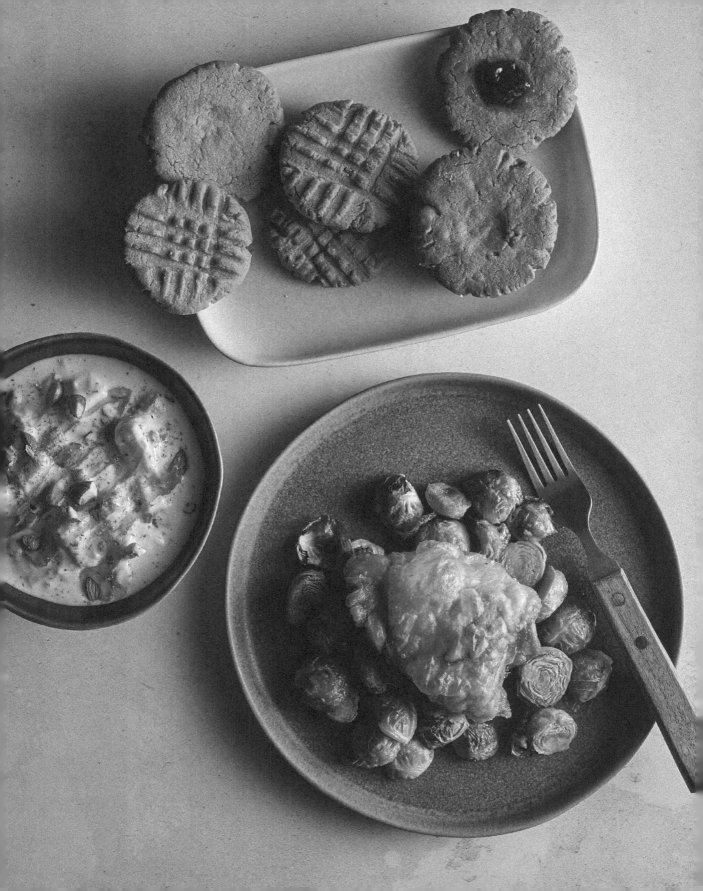

CONTENTS

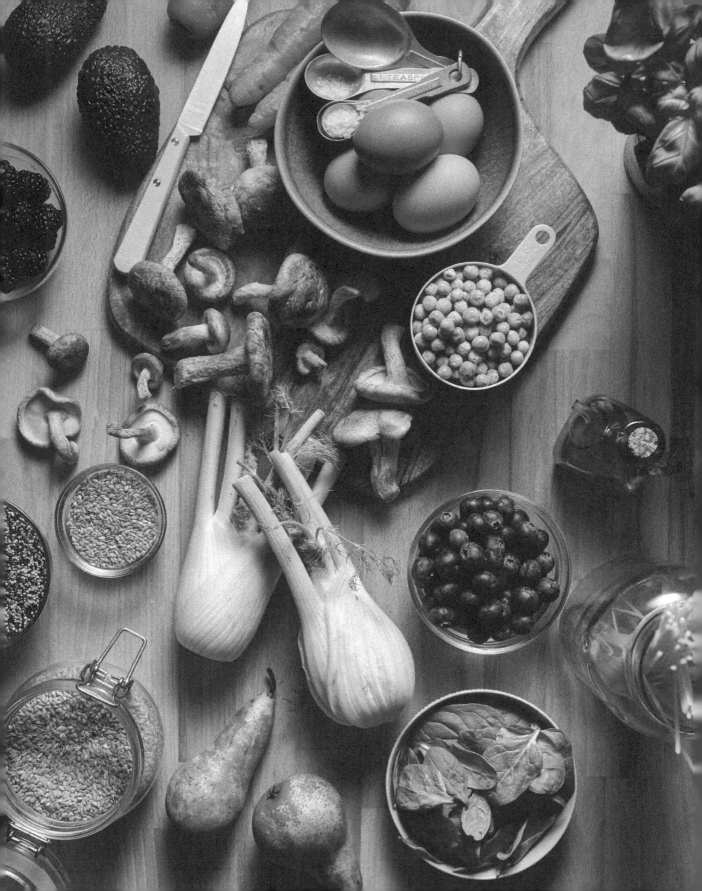

INTRODUCTION

Gastroesophageal reflux disease (GERD) affects millions of North Americans, and I used to be one of them. I was fortunate enough in my teenage years to resolve the condition through diet and lifestyle changes. Even though I didn't really know what was going on back then, I knew the persistent heartburn and reflux had to stop. I'm willing to bet that many of you feel the same, and I'm here to help.

My name is Andy De Santis and I'm a registered dietitian in private practice from Toronto, Canada. I understand just how much uncertainty around triggering heartburn and reflux can detract from your quality of life and enjoyment of food. I've taught my clients the diet and lifestyle fundamentals that contribute to fewer symptoms and a better quality of life in their fight against GERD. I'm happy to say that I'm here to put you on that same path. Using the best available scientific evidence, I'm going to nudge you toward a style of eating that helps put your health back in your hands.

I fully appreciate that you've purchased this book because you deal with some form of acid reflux, heartburn, GERD, or lower esophageal sphincter dysfunction and you want to start fighting back. It's important for you to understand that although these conditions were previously considered something that only older adults dealt with, the statistics show that they are becoming increasingly common in younger adults. If you fall into that category, know that you aren't alone.

I'm actually a great example of the trend—and coming out the other side of it. Having dealt with the pain and discomfort of acid reflux in young adulthood, I know just how much of a burden it can become. My personal experiences taught me how big a difference simple yet impactful changes to your behaviors and food choices can make when it comes to improving your symptoms. My professional experiences echo that sentiment. I've worked with a great number of people dealing with various extents of GERD, acid reflux, and heartburn over the years, and I've overseen great improvements in these patients' symptoms and overall health.

The information provided in this book will lead to meaningful changes in your overall health and quality of life.

The level of research I have put into this book has further enhanced my understanding, and suffice to say all those tidbits of knowledge are made available to you in the pages to come. I fully explore the best scientific evidence about preventing, managing, and fighting back against heartburn, acid reflex, and related conditions. This guidance is brought to life in both delicious and practical fashion with an array of five-ingredient recipes that will change the way you think about GERD-friendly eating.

I want you to dive in with the confidence that every consideration has been taken to ensure that the information provided in this book will lead to meaningful changes in your overall health and quality of life. From there you can explore the 100 recipes knowing that delicious GERD-friendly meals are possible.

Let's get started!

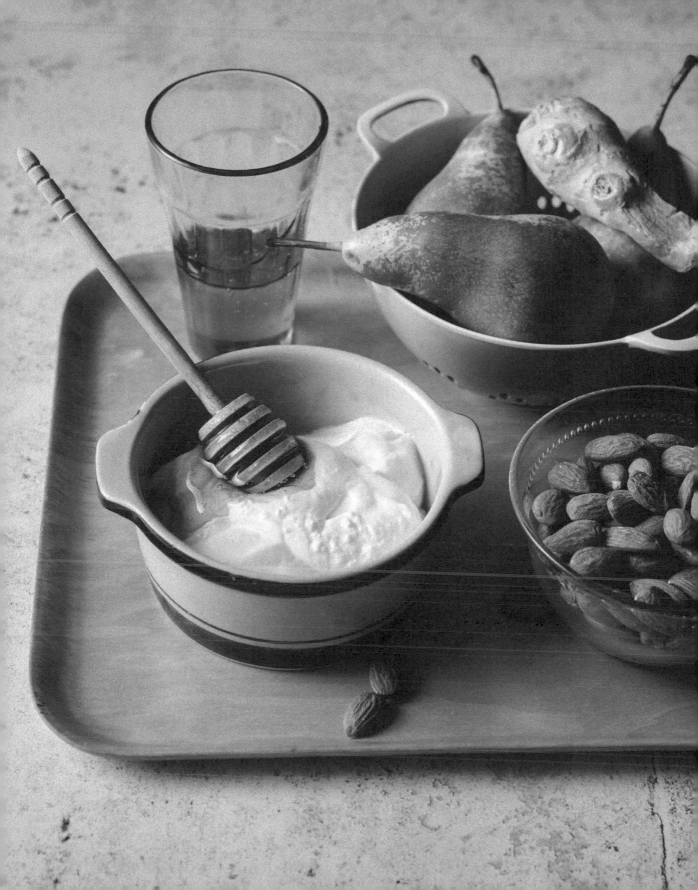

COD AND FENNEL PACKETS, PAGE 76

1

A Fresh Approach to Healing Acid Reflux

The first step to managing your acid reflux is to better understand what may be causing it and why. For some people, this question may be easier to answer than others. In the sections to come, I will offer information that will give you a clearer image of what's actually going on and what you can do about it.

Although it's quite possible that you may have already spoken about GERD with at least one member of your healthcare team, don't worry if you haven't yet. The goal of this chapter is to provide you with a solid understanding of the causes, symptoms, and management strategies for acid reflux.

On that note, let's start things off by defining what we mean by acid reflux and GERD, terms that are often used interchangeably even though they aren't quite the same thing.

What Is Acid Reflux?

Acid reflux is defined as the backward flow of gastric acid from the stomach through the lower esophageal sphincter (LES) and into the esophagus. This tends to cause the infamous burning sensation known as heartburn, among other unpleasant consequences such as belching, coughing, and wheezing. According to the American College of Gastroenterology (ACG), more than 60 million Americans experience heartburn at least once a month, and it has a lot to do with issues in how the LES is functioning.

The LES is a circular muscle that is responsible for opening and closing the passage between the esophagus and the stomach that ultimately allows food to travel from the mouth to the stomach. This muscle tightens and closes to prevent stomach acid from moving back up the esophagus, the tube that connects the mouth to the stomach. Problems arise when the sphincter no longer seals as tightly as it used to, which can occur for a number of reasons that I'll outline later in this chapter.

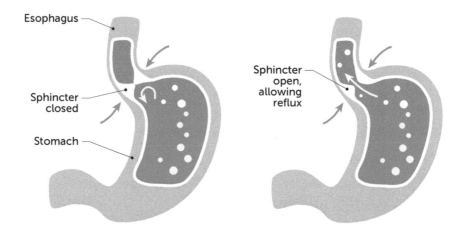

An isolated incident of acid reflux is unpleasant, but when it starts to occur regularly, you may have a bigger problem on your hands. Frequent heartburn, belching, and stomach pain when lying down are all signs of a more severe condition known as gastroesophageal reflux disease (GERD). The ACG guidelines define GERD as "symptoms or complications resulting from the reflux of gastric contents into the esophagus or beyond, into the oral cavity (including larynx) or lung."

If you've been formally diagnosed with GERD or suspect that you might have it based on this description, it's important to seek medical care and know that you aren't alone in doing so. GERD is considered among the most common illnesses in the world, with about one in six North Americans suffering from it.

Traditionally, GERD was thought of as a condition that impacted only populations in the 50-plus age bracket, but the latest data shows that people in younger age groups, especially ages 30 to 39, are being diagnosed more frequently. This is at least a reflection of less-than-ideal diet and lifestyle habits, a topic we explore further in the pages to come.

Some people may also experience what is known as laryngopharyngeal reflux (LPR), in which the stomach acid moves farther up the digestive tract toward the larynx, or "voice box," leading to symptoms that may more closely resemble a sore throat and, as a result, may be more likely to be missed or undiagnosed. Treatments for GERD and LPR range widely and may include medicine and even surgery in the most severe cases. Dietary and lifestyle choices, as you will see in the sections to come, can also play an important role in managing symptoms and improving your quality of life.

The Root Causes and Symptoms of GERD and LPR

The functionality of your LES can be compromised by a number of factors, including aging, a weak dietary pattern, inactivity, and certain physical characteristics, such as weak abdominal muscles (including due to a hernia), which may make you more susceptible to GERD. Significant changes to the body, such as pregnancy or rapid weight gain due to other factors, may also temporarily increase your risk of GERD-related symptoms. Lifestyle factors, such as drinking, smoking, wearing tight-fitting clothing, eating too close to bedtime,

WHEN SHOULD I SEE A DOCTOR?

Diet and lifestyle modifications can play an important role in managing acid reflux, but severe and persistent symptoms often require further medical attention.

Some people may experience symptom improvement in a matter of weeks once the appropriate diet and lifestyle strategies are employed. Others, though, may be at a more advanced stage where these strategies need to be combined with diligent medical observation and care.

Anyone experiencing severe or frequent symptoms, such as intolerable chest pain or coughing at night that interferes with sleep, should see their doctor immediately. Those who have diligently applied the guidance in this book for a number of weeks but see

no symptom improvement should also seek further medical care.

Quick questions to ask yourself:

- Have the symptoms lasted more than two weeks even with dietary changes and over-the-counter medication?
- Is the frequency or severity worsening?
- Is it affecting your sleep?
- Have you lost your appetite as a result of the symptoms?

If the answer to any of these questions is yes, it's not a bad idea to check with an ear, nose, and throat specialist (ENT) as soon as possible.

and the types of food you consume, also play a role. The more of these risk factors that are present, the more likely an individual could suffer from GERD, LPR, or both.

Aside from being both unpleasant and painful, chronic reflux comes with long-term risks. When the cells of the esophagus are chronically exposed to stomach acid, they can be damaged and transformed, leading to a condition known as Barrett's esophagus. Although not common, Barrett's esophagus can increase your risk of esophageal cancer, and it should not be taken lightly. Similarly, severe cases of LPR that are left unmanaged may increase one's risk of bronchitis, pneumonitis, and damage to the tissues of the throat and voice box.

The Relationship Between Food and Acid Reflux

Your best dietary defense against GERD involves a combination of avoiding foods that may cause your symptoms to flare up, and then embracing a core group of healthy, nutrient-dense foods that will optimize your health and the functioning of your digestive system.

Certain types of foods may either directly contribute to symptoms by aggravating an already sensitive esophagus or may indirectly contribute to further acid reflux through a variety of means, including relaxing your lower esophageal sphincter or creating additional pressure in your abdominal area that may contribute to forcing stomach acid upward. Triggers for acid reflux may vary widely from person to person, so diligent observation is important to understand how certain types of food affect your symptoms. There are, however, a core group of foods that GERD sufferers tend to report most frequently as triggers.

Because they tend to be slightly more acidic than most other foods, citrus fruits such as oranges, grapefruit, and lemons (and their juices) and tomato-based products such as sauces and ketchup may not be as well tolerated by those with GERD. When it comes to issues of the digestive tract, garlic and onions are also generally known as repeat offenders; they may contribute to gas and bloating while also potentially increasing reflux risk by relaxing the

LES. Very spicy foods are often identified as reflux triggers and may irritate an already-damaged esophagus. And dietary patterns characterized by high intake of meats, oils, and fatty or fried foods tend to increase the risk of acid reflux because they slow the rate at which food empties from the stomach.

On the other end of the spectrum, fish and high-fiber foods such as vegetables, legumes, nuts, seeds, and whole grains are all foods that I feel are particularly important to ensure that your dietary pattern is strong. A 2005 study in the *British Medical Journal* found that high-fiber diets were associated with a reduced risk of GERD-related symptoms. This is partially due to the fact that when dietary fiber is low, food does not move as quickly or efficiently through your digestive tract, which may increase your risk of reflux and other gastrointestinal issues. Additionally, a 2017 study in the *Journal of the American Medical Association* found that Mediterranean-style diets—which emphasize protein from largely plant-based sources such as legumes, nuts, and seeds as well as some seafood—were at least as effective if not more effective than medication when it came to symptom reduction in a group of patients with LPR.

When considering a GERD-friendly diet, it's also worth knowing a bit about FODMAPs: short-chain carbohydrates that are poorly absorbed in the small intestine, causing gas that can contribute to intra-abdominal pressure. A 2017 study in the *American Journal of Gastroenterology* and a 2014 study in the *Clinical Nutritional Journal* found some evidence that lower-FODMAP diets may help those living with GERD, heartburn, and acid reflux. Things like bread, pasta, garlic, and cow's milk are higher-FODMAP foods, while oatmeal, gluten-free bread/pasta, and almond milk are lower-FODMAP foods. The recipes in this book focus on foods that tend to be lower in FODMAPs.

Please keep in mind that if you suffer from irritable bowel syndrome (IBS) beyond just GERD, reflux, or heartburn, you should consider seeking out the help of a health professional to guide you further on how to make the most of a lower-FODMAP style of eating.

Food Tables

The following are helpful summaries of foods to minimize and foods you can enjoy without worrying that they will trigger a flare-up. It's important to keep in mind that the "minimize these foods" list in particular consists of the foods that are most likely to be acid reflux triggers, and they have been excluded from the recipes in this book. Even so, there are people who can manage their GERD while still eating foods from this list. If you find that you can enjoy a particular food symptom-free, you do not need to discontinue its use.

MINIMIZE THESE FOODS

Food or Food Group	Noteworthy Information
Alcoholic beverages	May relax LES
Butter and oil	Be mindful of amount used; can significantly increase fat content of meal and contribute to reflux risk in some
Caffeine	Stimulant, may relax LES
Carbonated beverages	May increase abdominal pressure
Chiles, peppers, hot sauce	Common reflux triggers
Chocolate	Stimulant, common reflux cause
Citrus fruits and juices	Acidic, may irritate esophagus
Cream sauces	High in fat, may increase risk of reflux
Curry	Spicy varieties common reflux triggers
Dairy, full-fat or medium-fat (2 percent)	Avoid high-fat dairy such as butter, cheese, whole milk, full-fat yogurt and sour cream, and cream—if you use, use sparingly
Fried foods	Common heartburn and reflux trigger
Fruit	Acidic fruits, fruits not listed on page 8, pineapple, citrus
Garlic	Common reflux trigger, high-FODMAP
Meat, beef	Avoid fatty cuts
Meat, pork	Avoid fatty cuts
Onion	Common reflux trigger, high-FODMAP
Pepper, black	Common reflux trigger
Peppermint	Common reflux trigger
Pineapple	Acidic, may irritate some
Potato chips and French fries	High fat content may irritate some if consumed in large quantities
Spicy food	Common reflux trigger
Tea	Common reflux trigger
Tomatoes and tomato-based sauces	Including salsa, pizza sauce, and pasta sauce—may be irritating for some due to acidity

ENJOY WITH GUSTO

Food or Food Group	Noteworthy Information
Avocado	Excellent source of soluble fiber and healthy fats; high in FODMAPs
Banana	Contains soluble fiber, good for digestive health; green varieties are low in FODMAPs
Beef, extra-lean cuts	Less than 15 percent fat
Berries	High in fiber, vitamins, and minerals; low-FODMAP
Breads and crackers	Preferably whole grain for more fiber
Canned lentils	High source of soluble fiber; ½ cup serving is low-FODMAP
Cheese	Nonfat—lactose-free if sensitive to FODMAPs
Citrus zest	Citrus flavor, less acidic
Corn	All kinds, including cornmeal—avoid if sensitive to FODMAPs
Eggs	Good source of protein and vitamin D
Fennel	May improve stomach's digestive function
Fish and shellfish	All types, minimize fried
Fish sauce	Great way to add umami flavor
Flaxseeds	High in soluble fiber and anti-inflammatory omega-3 fatty acids
Ginger	Fresh or ground
Herbs and spices	All but peppers, chiles, and mint
Legumes	Chickpeas, beans, peas, etc.
Maple syrup	Low-FODMAP sweetener
Melon	Cantaloupe, honeydew, or watermelon
Milk	Nonfat, 1 percent, soy, almond, or rice
Miso	Adds flavor
Mushrooms	All varieties
Oatmeal	High in soluble fiber, contributes to improved digestive health
Olive oil	1 to 2 tablespoons daily
Pasta	Tomato sauce is a trigger in some; gluten-free pasta if you have a gluten sensitivity
Pear	Good source of fiber, high-FODMAP
Popcorn	Preferably air-popped
Poultry	Skinless, not fried
Poultry broth or stock	Homemade is best
Pumpkin seeds	High in fiber, high in protein, and support gut health; low-FODMAP
Sea salt	This is not a low-sodium diet; however, if you have a history of hypertension, reduce the salt

Food or Food Group	Noteworthy Information
Seaweed	Antioxidant-rich snack food, supports the growth of healthy gut bacteria
Soy sauce	Great way to add flavor; choose gluten-free if needed
Sugar	Moderate amounts of brown or white sugar add flavor
Tempeh	Plant-based protein source, contains probiotics
Tofu	Excellent protein source for vegetarian meals
Vegetables, green	High in fiber; broccoli, zucchini, spinach, and kale are lower-FODMAP
Vegetables, root (tubers)	Carrots, potatoes, sweet potato, turnips, etc.; noted exception: onions
Yogurt	Low-fat, plain, nonfat, Greek—lactose-free if lactose intolerant, probiotic for strong gut health

Dietary and Lifestyle Changes to Soothe Acid Reflux

In addition to focusing on specific types of foods, there are a number of broader dietary and lifestyle changes you can introduce to reduce your risk of experiencing GERD-related symptoms.

- **EAT YOUR LAST MEAL OF THE DAY EARLIER.** I regularly ask my clients how long they wait between taking their last bite of food at night and then going to bed or lying down on the couch. Multiple studies show that the likelihood of reflux symptoms is much higher in those who quickly transition from dinner to bed. According to a 2016 study in the Baltimore journal *Medicine,* the risk of stomach cancer is also higher in these groups of people. One of the biggest reasons is that gravity is no longer in your favor. When you are upright, the muscles of your stomach and gravity are working in the same direction; this is not the case when you are lying down.

- **KEEP YOUR HEAD ELEVATED WHILE YOU SLEEP.** In addition to avoiding meals close to bedtime, elevating the head of your bed by four to six inches while sleeping is commonly recommended to GERD sufferers to reduce the risk of reflux overnight.

- **QUIT SMOKING.** The ill health effects of smoking are well known and expand into the realm of GERD by increasing the production of stomach acid and weakening the LES, which may make you more prone to reflux and other GERD-related symptoms.

- **WEAR LOOSE-FITTING CLOTHING.** We all have that pair of pants or T-shirt that does not fit the way it used to. Unfortunately, tight clothing may cause more than just discomfort. The additional pressure it applies on the stomach can increase your risk of suffering GERD-related symptoms.

- **EAT SMALLER, MORE FREQUENT MEALS.** Because people living with GERD and related symptoms tend to have a lower esophageal sphincter that is not functioning optimally, you want to make that muscle's job as easy as possible. One of the ways to do this is by refraining from very large meals and instead focusing on smaller meals and snacks throughout the day.

- **KEEP A FOOD AND SYMPTOM DIARY.** One of the key things to keep in mind with acid reflux and GERD is that different people respond to different foods in different ways. There are common trigger foods that may not bother you, and you may be troubled by foods that are not often considered triggers. One step to take to learn more about your symptoms is to keep a food and symptom diary.

ALTERNATIVE SOURCES OF GERD RELIEF

In addition to the dietary and lifestyle changes discussed so far, there is a growing body of evidence that suggests that alternative therapies and even certain supplements may play an important role in managing GERD symptoms in some people. The alternative strategies have good evidence to support them but are not yet considered mainstream treatment approaches. As such, you should first discuss their suitability with your healthcare professional before pursuing them.

ACUPUNCTURE. A 2010 study in the *Chinese Journal of Integrative Medicine* found that individuals with GERD who were treated with acupuncture at the CV12, ST36, and PC6 trigger points experienced a reduction in reflux symptoms. A 2014 paper in the *Journal of Clinical Gastroenterology* also confirmed the potential of acupuncture to aid those suffering from frequent acid reflux.

ACTIVE BREATHING EXERCISES. Breath training, which is often done as a part of yoga practice and can be pursued independently, is often considered an effective tool for stress reduction and management. The lower esophageal sphincter is surrounded by muscles of the diaphragm, which are the ones most often engaged in breathing exercises. When the muscles of the diaphragm are more actively engaged, the risk for GERD and reflux is lessened, as demonstrated in a 2012 study in the *American Journal of Gastroenterology*.

MELATONIN SUPPLEMENTATION. Melatonin is often considered the "sleep hormone" because it plays a role in modulating your biological clock, also known as your circadian rhythm. It is one of the top-selling supplements on the market, and there is growing interest around its potential to help those living with GERD. In fact, a 2010 study in the journal *BMC Gastroenterology* found that melatonin supplementation in combination with standard medical therapy helped more than medical therapy alone.

PSYLLIUM FIBER. Psyllium fiber is a special type of plant fiber often sold in supplemental form or added to products such as breakfast cereals for its digestive health benefits. Often recommended for the treatment of IBS, constipation, and some forms of diarrhea, psyllium fiber is also known to help with both blood sugar and blood cholesterol levels. What intrigues me, however, is a 2018 study in the *Journal of Evidence-Based Integrative Medicine* that found that psyllium actually helped reduce the symptoms of GERD in individuals dealing with constipation.

The Five-Ingredient Fix

If you are living with GERD, you may feel as though every meal is a battle. The goal of the next few sections is to show that you can fight back with five ingredients or fewer to create delicious meals.

The recipes in this book were designed specifically to include commonly available ingredients that will play a big role in improving the quality of your diet and overall health while reducing your GERD symptoms. The recipe ingredients are as GERD-friendly as possible, and their easy preparations ensure a transition with less prep, minimal cleanup, and simpler trips to the grocery store. Most of the recipes call for small amounts of sea salt and olive oil (or olive oil cooking spray), two GERD-friendly ingredients that are not counted toward the five-ingredient total.

Keeping in mind that the goal of these recipes is to make your life as easy as possible, some of the recipes call for convenient ingredients that may be canned, packaged, jarred, frozen, or bottled. When it comes to packaged products, whether for use in the recipes in this book or for daily use or preference, be mindful of any ingredients that may be potential triggers for you. This will, of course, require you to have a level of understanding of potential irritant foods and then to use that knowledge when reviewing the ingredient lists of packaged products.

Products with smaller ingredient lists simplify this process. Super common ingredients, such as garlic and onions, can be bothersome for people living with GERD or digestive issues, so if you find yourself in this boat, keep a watchful eye. Since very fatty meals can slow down stomach emptying and increase the risk of reflux, be wary when choosing from products high in fat and go for ones that have less fat. Anything that appears to be fatty, fried, or spicy, as a general rule, should be used with caution. And choose products that are higher in fiber whenever possible.

Stocking Your Pantry and Kitchen

In any five-ingredient cookbook, convenience is king. That's exactly why a good number of the recipes in this book use nonperishable ingredients widely available at most grocery stores. As far as kitchen equipment is concerned, the vast majority of the recipes can be put together with common utensils and cookware you probably already have. Let's take a closer look at what you'll need to succeed.

PANTRY ESSENTIALS

High-fiber, plant-based eating tends to be the best direction to go for optimal health and GERD management. The pantry essentials I've selected emphasize these principles. Whenever possible, I offer replacements for common trigger foods and take FODMAPs into consideration for those who may be affected by them. Here are some ingredients to have handy:

- Almonds, chopped
- Chia seeds
- Cinnamon
- Cumin
- Ginger, ground
- Honey
- Maple syrup, pure
- Olive oil (and olive oil cooking spray)
- Sea salt
- Soy sauce, low-sodium
- Thyme, dried

KITCHEN TOOLS

I've made it a point to ensure that you won't need anything too funky to bring the recipes in this book to life. I want them to be as accessible as possible. If I had to pick the top 12 most important pieces of cookware and/or kitchen utensils you will need, they'd be these:

- Baking sheets and pans suitable for stove-top grilling, various sizes
- Blender and/or food processor
- Cutting boards (at least two)
- Glass or plastic airtight containers for storage
- Knife set

- Parchment paper
- Saucepans, various sizes
- Skillet, large nonstick
- Soup pot
- Steaming basket
- Vegetable peeler
- Wooden spoons

MAKING THE SWITCH TO AN ACID-FREE LIFESTYLE

The cliché of adjusting the way you eat being a "lifestyle change" is never truer than when it comes to your fight against GERD and acid reflux. I say this because a great deal of what you need to do to minimize your risk of symptoms goes well beyond what you choose to eat.

So far, I've reviewed some of the major considerations to ease your transition into what I call an "acid-free lifestyle," but we aren't quite done yet. Consider this section a friendly reminder of what we've discussed so far and the "icing on the cake" to the journey you are about to take.

SHARE YOUR GOALS. One of the fundamental pillars of behavior change theory is sharing your goals with those closest to you. This does not necessarily mean telling everyone about your diet and lifestyle changes. Rather, it means confiding in those closest to you (family, spouse, best friend) about the changes you hope to make and why you are making them. This will provide you with an extra layer of support and accountability, which is invaluable during the initial period of change when it can be the most challenging.

SHIFT YOUR EATING PATTERN. I've already established the complete and utter importance of not eating too close to bedtime when you are living with GERD. For some, this simply may mean omitting your evening snack, but for others it may require a much more significant commitment to changing daily routines. Those of you who have after-work events, work late, or work out in the evening may have grown accustomed to late-night meals and will be able to shake this habit only if extra consideration is made to accommodate the change.

EAT OUT LESS. If you eat out more than two or three times per week, I want to challenge you to reduce your meals out by 50 percent. Although not impossible, it is in most cases challenging to eat what we consider a GERD-friendly meal when you are eating out. This is largely due to the amount of sauces, spices, and other ingredients used in restaurants. And, of course, I want you to eat as many delicious recipes from this book as possible as well!

The Recipes in This Book

If you are anything like me, seeing a recipe that requires 20-plus ingredients makes heartburn even worse. That certainly is not the goal with this book. These recipes have been specifically crafted with all the evidence surrounding nutrition and acid reflux that we've discussed so far. In other words, these recipes are as GERD-friendly as they can be.

I have provided you with a wide array of recipes that you can mix and match as you see fit. And the best part? Aside from our two main pantry staples, salt and olive oil, all recipes require five or fewer ingredients.

Although we have vastly different needs as to the total amount of calories we eat on a daily basis, I tried to create the recipes in keeping with the notion that people living with GERD are best served by having multiple small meals and snacks per day. Keep that in mind if you are wondering why the serving sizes look smaller than you might be used to—this is intentional.

Each recipe is designed to create between two and four servings. Most recipes are stand-alone meals; however, snacks, sauces, stocks, and condiments are also included and can be incorporated as you see fit. To help with your meal planning, the recipes contain addition labels: low-FODMAP, vegan or vegetarian, and gluten-free. You will also find tips at the end of each recipe to help you with selecting ingredients, substitutions, and ways to boost the flavor of the recipe or modify it for batch cooking.

I appreciate how challenging it can be to make and commit to a dietary change, especially in the early stages. I made sure no stone was left unturned in creating a comprehensive yet easy-to-use library of recipes to help you bring the guidance you've read so far to life.

I truly hope you enjoy them.

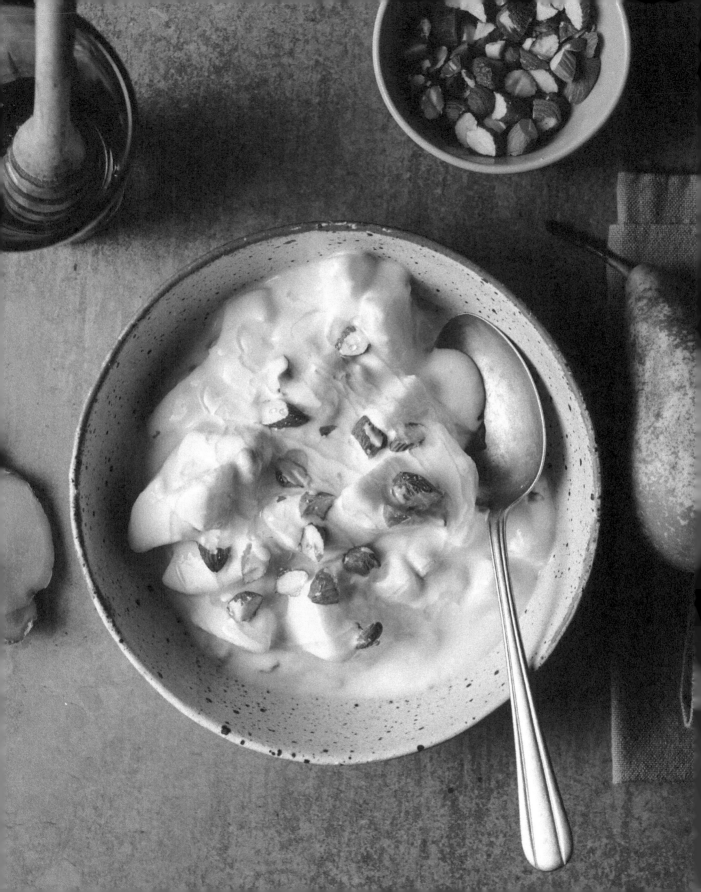

Breakfast

If you're always on the go in the morning, then these overnight oats are a lifesaver. They provide a hearty breakfast you can make ahead and just grab and go. The addition of freshly grated ginger helps soothe GERD, as can the alkaline nature of oats. If you're gluten-sensitive or avoiding FODMAPs, make sure the oats you select are specifically labeled gluten-free.

OVERNIGHT CINNAMON OATS

SERVES: 1 · **PREP TIME:** 5 minutes, plus overnight soaking

LOW-FODMAP
VEGETARIAN

½ cup skim milk
½ cup old-fashioned oats
½ teaspoon grated fresh ginger
½ teaspoon cinnamon

1. Combine all the ingredients in a jar or a sealable container. Mix well. Refrigerate overnight.

2. Stir before eating.

SUBSTITUTION TIP: Make these oats vegan by replacing the skim milk with a low-fat nondairy milk such as plain almond milk or plain rice milk. Add flavor by adding up to 2 tablespoons of raisins if they don't aggravate your GERD.

PER SERVING: *Calories: 195; Total fat: 3g; Sodium: 52mg; Carbohydrates: 34g; Fiber: 5g; Protein: 9g*

This breakfast comes together in a flash, and it's easy to double or triple the recipe to serve the whole family. Adjust the amount of honey to your preferred level of sweetness. This bowl is especially delicious with fresh, local, in-season pears, although you can also use canned pears (in juice). If you do buy pears in juice, opt for organic pears in 100 percent juice.

GINGERED YOGURT AND PEAR BOWLS

SERVES: 1 • **PREP TIME:** 5 minutes

GLUTEN-FREE
VEGETARIAN

½ **cup plain nonfat Greek yogurt**
2 **tablespoons honey**
½ **teaspoon grated fresh ginger**
1 **pear, peeled, cored, and chopped**
1 **tablespoon chopped almonds**

1. In a small bowl, mix together the yogurt, honey (to taste), and ginger.

2. Stir in the pear and chopped almonds.

FLAVOR BOOST: Replace the honey with an equal amount of pure maple syrup and add ¼ teaspoon of nutmeg.

PER SERVING: Calories: 313; Total fat: 4g; Sodium: 47mg; Carbohydrates: 62g; Fiber: 5g; Protein: 13g

Smoothies make the perfect on-the-go breakfasts, and chia is a good source of fiber. When chia is mixed with liquid, it creates a gel that can help fill you up while soothing an irritated digestive tract. The trick to a delicious smoothie is making sure the ingredients you use are very cold. Add ice cubes to thicken and chill your smoothie further. Feel free to substitute any berry for blueberries in this smoothie.

BLUEBERRY, SPINACH, AND CHIA SMOOTHIE

SERVES: 1 • **PREP TIME:** 5 minutes

GLUTEN-FREE
LOW-FODMAP
VEGAN

2 cups baby spinach
1½ cups low-fat or plain nondairy milk
1 cup fresh or frozen blueberries
1 tablespoon chia seeds
½ teaspoon cinnamon

In a blender, combine all the ingredients. Blend until smooth.

————

BATCH IT: This smoothie keeps quite well in the fridge for up to 3 days, so you can double or triple the batch. Before serving on each subsequent day, give it a few pulses in the blender.

————

PER SERVING: *Calories: 314; Total fat: 7g; Sodium: 259mg; Carbohydrates: 46g; Fiber: 12g; Protein: 18g*

This smoothie is naturally thick, and ginger, avocado, and bananas make it delicious and perfect for calming your acid reflux. The alkaline nature of bananas and avocados is especially helpful for soothing GERD, although you want to avoid overdoing it with avocados due to the fat content. Try to limit avocado servings to a quarter to a half of an avocado. If you don't have fresh ginger, add ½ teaspoon of ground ginger from the spice rack instead.

BANANA-AVO SMOOTHIE

SERVES: 1 · **PREP TIME:** 5 minutes

GLUTEN-FREE
VEGETARIAN

1½ cups low-fat milk or
    plain nondairy milk
    such as almond milk
1 banana
¼ avocado, peeled
    and pitted
1 tablespoon pure
    maple syrup
½ teaspoon grated
    fresh ginger

In a blender, combine all the ingredients. Blend until smooth.

INGREDIENT TIP: Want a thick, milkshake-like smoothie? Freeze the banana (unpeeled) before you toss it in the smoothie.

PER SERVING: Calories: 381; Total fat: 11g; Sodium: 187mg; Carbohydrates: 61g; Fiber: 6g; Protein: 14g

Whether you top these pancakes with pure maple syrup or Gingered Red Applesauce (page 137) or enjoy them on their own, these are sure to satisfy even the pickiest of pancake lovers. You can save cooked pancakes in a zip-top bag in the refrigerator and reheat them in the microwave for additional meals. With alkaline pumpkin and soothing fresh ginger, this recipe is great for GERD.

PUMPKIN PANCAKES

SERVES: 4 · **PREP TIME:** 5 minutes · **COOK TIME:** 10 minutes

VEGETARIAN

4 large eggs, beaten
1 cup pumpkin puree
  (not pumpkin pie filling)
½ cup whole-wheat flour
1 teaspoon grated
  fresh ginger
Nonstick cooking spray

1. In a medium bowl, whisk together the eggs, pumpkin, flour, and ginger.

2. Spray a large nonstick skillet with nonstick cooking spray and place over medium-high heat. Once the pan is hot, spoon the batter ¼ cup at a time onto the skillet.

3. Cook until bubbles form on the top, about 3 minutes. Flip and cook 3 minutes more.

SUBSTITUTION TIP: If you need this to be gluten-free, replace the whole-wheat flour with gluten-free oat flour.

PER SERVING: *Calories: 143; Total fat: 5g; Sodium: 74mg; Carbohydrates: 16g; Fiber: 4g; Protein: 9g*

These are so easy to make, and you can use fresh herbs or a little bit of crumbled turkey bacon to jazz up the original recipe. While most people with GERD do well with avocado because of its alkaline nature, if you are sensitive to FODMAPs, you'll want to skip this recipe.

BAKED EGG AND AVOCADO

SERVES: 2 • **PREP TIME:** 10 minutes • **COOK TIME:** 15 minutes

GLUTEN-FREE
VEGETARIAN

1 avocado, halved lengthwise, peeled and pitted
2 large eggs
Pinch sea salt

1. Preheat the oven to 400°F.

2. Place the avocado halves cut-side up on a baking sheet. Use a metal spoon to scoop out a little bit of the avocado from the center to enlarge the pit area, which is where you'll put the eggs. Reserve the scooped-out avocado for another purpose.

3. Carefully crack each egg into each avocado half.

4. Sprinkle the eggs and avocado halves with the sea salt.

5. Bake until the eggs are set, about 15 minutes.

INGREDIENT TIP: To remove the avocado half intact from the peel, use a large metal spoon and scoop the half out in one piece.

PER SERVING: Calories: 216; Total fat: 18g; Sodium: 117mg; Carbohydrates: 8g; Fiber: 6g; Protein: 8g

French toast is the perfect meal for lazy Sunday mornings, and it doesn't take long to whip this up—just 20 minutes. Serve it plain, sprinkled with a bit of powdered sugar, or top with pure maple syrup.

GINGER CRÈME BRÛLÉE FRENCH TOAST

SERVES: 4 · **PREP TIME:** 10 minutes · **COOK TIME:** 10 minutes

VEGETARIAN

4 large eggs, beaten
1 cup skim milk or
    nondairy milk
1 teaspoon grated
    fresh ginger
1 vanilla bean
4 slices bread
Nonstick cooking spray

1. In a large liquid measuring cup, whisk together the eggs, milk, and ginger.

2. Using a sharp knife, split the vanilla bean in half lengthwise. Use the tip of the knife to scrape the seeds from the center of the bean into the egg and milk mixture. Whisk again.

3. Pour the mixture into a shallow dish. Soak the bread in the egg mixture until the liquid is absorbed, about 3 minutes per side.

4. Spray a large nonstick skillet with nonstick cooking spray and place over medium-high heat. Once hot, add the bread and cook the French toast until the custard sets, about 4 minutes per side.

SUBSTITUTION TIP: To make this gluten-free, use gluten-free bread. To make it dairy-free, substitute a plain, nondairy milk such as rice milk.

PER SERVING: *Calories: 193; Total fat: 6g; Sodium: 257mg; Carbohydrates: 23g; Fiber: 3g; Protein: 12g*

Using veggies and eggs to make a quick scramble produces a hearty and fast breakfast with tons of flavor and alkaline, GERD-friendly greens. The scramble will keep well for about 3 days in the refrigerator, so it's also a great meal to make ahead and reheat in the microwave. To make this low-FODMAP, use oyster mushrooms, which are much lower in polyols than other mushrooms.

SPINACH AND MUSHROOM SCRAMBLE

SERVES: 4 · **PREP TIME:** 10 minutes · **COOK TIME:** 10 minutes

GLUTEN-FREE
VEGETARIAN

1 tablespoon olive oil
4 ounces mushrooms, sliced
2 cups baby spinach
4 large eggs
6 large egg whites
½ teaspoon sea salt

1. Place a large skillet over medium-high heat and add the olive oil. Once the oil begins to shimmer, add the mushrooms and cook, stirring occasionally, for 5 minutes, until browned.

2. Add the spinach and cook until wilted, about 1 minute more.

3. In a large bowl, whisk together the eggs and egg whites with the sea salt. Pour this over the vegetables.

4. Cook, stirring, until the eggs are set, about 3 minutes.

FLAVOR BOOST: Up the flavor of this dish by adding ½ teaspoon of dried thyme to the mushrooms as they cook.

PER SERVING: *Calories: 139; Total fat: 9g; Sodium: 463mg; Carbohydrates: 2g; Fiber: 1g; Protein: 13g*

Hash browns make a great side dish, or serve them with a fried egg on top for a delicious and quick meal. These hash browns have a hint of ginger in them, giving them phenomenal flavor that is also soothing to GERD.

SWEET POTATO HASH BROWNS

SERVES: 4 · **PREP TIME:** 10 minutes · **COOK TIME:** 15 minutes

GLUTEN-FREE

VEGAN

2 tablespoons olive oil
2 teaspoons grated
*   fresh ginger*
2 cups peeled and grated
*   sweet potatoes*
*   (about 2 potatoes)*
½ teaspoon sea salt

1. Place a large nonstick skillet over medium-high heat and add the olive oil.

2. In a bowl, mix together the ginger, sweet potatoes, and salt.

3. Once the oil is shimmering, spread the potatoes in an even layer on the bottom of the skillet.

4. Cook without stirring until the potatoes are browned on one side, about 5 minutes.

5. Use a spatula to turn the potatoes and cook to brown on the other side, about 5 minutes more.

SUBSTITUTION TIP: If you're sensitive to sweet potatoes due to their FODMAP content, replace them with an equal amount of grated carrots or grated white potato.

PER SERVING: *Calories: 131; Total fat: 7g; Sodium: 300mg; Carbohydrates: 16g; Fiber: 2g; Protein: 1g*

It's super easy to make your own breakfast sausage that's both FODMAP-friendly and GERD-friendly. Eat it on its own with a side of hash browns, use it in a sandwich, or scramble it with eggs for a fast and easy protein-packed breakfast. Be sure to stick to just one sausage patty as a serving so you don't put too much pressure on your LES.

SAGE-TURKEY BREAKFAST SAUSAGE

SERVES: 4 · **PREP TIME:** 10 minutes · **COOK TIME:** 15 minutes

GLUTEN-FREE
LOW-FODMAP

8 ounces 93 percent lean ground turkey
2 teaspoons ground sage
½ teaspoon dried thyme
½ teaspoon sea salt
1 tablespoon olive oil

1. In a large bowl, combine the ground turkey, sage, thyme, and salt. Mix well.

2. Form the mixture into 4 (2-ounce) patties.

3. Place a large nonstick skillet over medium-high heat and add the olive oil. Once the oil shimmers, add the patties and cook until browned on both sides, about 4 minutes per side.

BATCH IT: Because this sausage freezes so well, you can double or triple the batch, cook all the patties, and then freeze them in zip-top freezer bags for use during the week. They'll keep for up to 6 months in the freezer. Just thaw in the refrigerator before reheating in the microwave.

PER SERVING: *Calories: 112; Total fat: 8g; Sodium: 333mg; Carbohydrates: <1g; Fiber: <1g; Protein: 11g*

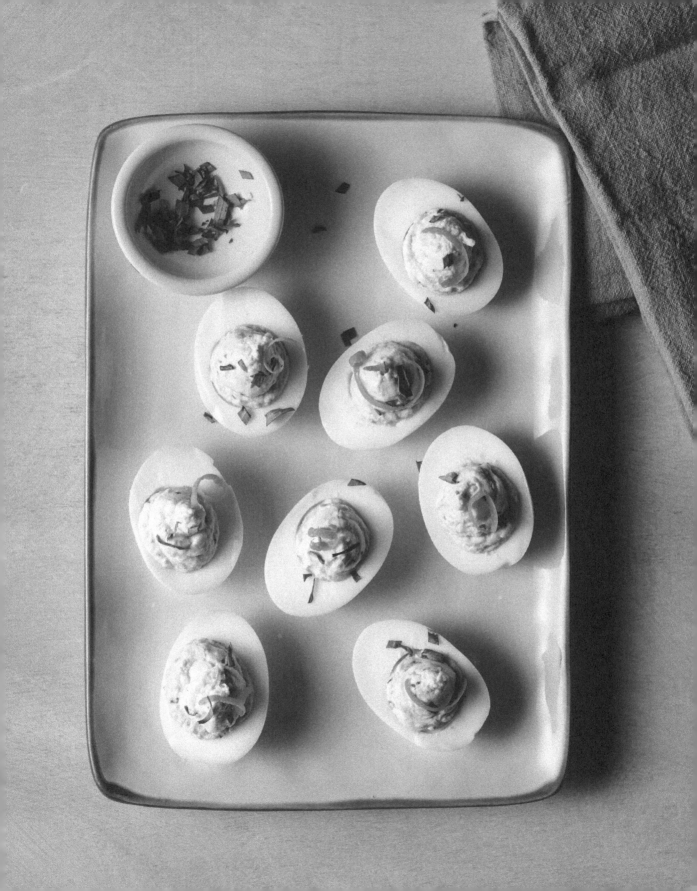

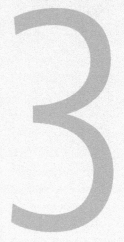

Sides and Snacks

Guacamole is a delicious sandwich spread. You can also use it to top eggs, fish, or meat or as a delicious dip for alkaline veggies such as jicama, carrots, or celery sticks. Because you don't add any acid to this guacamole and acid is what keeps avocados from turning brown, this is best when made shortly before you eat it. If you don't need six servings, you can halve the recipe.

GUACAMOLE

SERVES: 6 · **PREP TIME:** 10 minutes

GLUTEN-FREE
VEGETARIAN

2 avocados, peeled, pitted, and chopped
¼ cup chopped fresh cilantro
2 tablespoons fat-free plain Greek yogurt
½ teaspoon ground cumin
½ teaspoon grated lime zest
½ teaspoon sea salt or to taste

Combine all the ingredients in a medium bowl. Mash and mix with a fork until the avocados are mashed and the ingredients are well blended.

———————————

INGREDIENT TIP: Choose avocados that have a little bit of give when you press on the skin with your thumb but not so much that your finger feels as if it will poke through. You can also remove the stem of the avocado. The flesh underneath should be green.

———————————

PER SERVING: Calories: 101; Total fat: 9g; Sodium: 202mg; Carbohydrates: 5g; Fiber: 4g; Protein: 2g

Deviled eggs make a great snack or even a light meal. Orange zest and tarragon add flavor without acid, while the avocado brings alkalinity to the dish and provides a creamy texture to the egg yolks. These will keep for about 2 days in the refrigerator. Wrap them tightly with plastic wrap to keep the avocados from oxidizing and browning.

AVOCADO DEVILED EGGS

SERVES: 4 · **PREP TIME:** 10 minutes

GLUTEN-FREE
VEGETARIAN

4 large hardboiled eggs, peeled and sliced in half lengthwise
2 tablespoons fat-free plain Greek yogurt
½ avocado, peeled, pitted, and mashed
1 teaspoon orange zest
¼ cup chopped fresh tarragon
½ teaspoon sea salt

1. Use a spoon to scoop the egg yolks from the whites. Put the egg yolks in a small bowl and put the whites, cut-side up, on a platter.

2. Add the yogurt, avocado, orange zest, tarragon, and salt to the egg yolks. Mash with a fork and mix.

3. Spoon or pipe the mixture into the egg halves.

INGREDIENT TIP: To hard-boil eggs, put them in the bottom of a large pot in a single layer. Cover with at least 1 inch of cold water and put on the stove. Turn the heat to medium-high and bring the water to a boil. When the water boils, turn off the heat and leave the pan on the burner. Cover the pan and let the eggs sit in the water for 14 minutes. Using tongs, remove the eggs and plunge them into ice water to stop the cooking process.

PER SERVING: *Calories: 123; Total fat: 9g; Sodium: 358mg; Carbohydrates: 4g; Fiber: 2g; Protein: 8g*

Fennel is known to soothe GERD. It has an anise-like flavor (think licorice) that has a delicious caramelized flavor and aroma when roasted.

ROASTED FENNEL

SERVES: 4 · **PREP TIME:** 10 minutes · **COOK TIME:** 40 minutes

GLUTEN-FREE
LOW-FODMAP
VEGAN

2 fennel bulbs, cored and cut into pieces
2 tablespoons olive oil
½ teaspoon sea salt
½ teaspoon grated lemon zest

1. Preheat the oven to 400°F.

2. In a large bowl, toss the fennel with the olive oil and salt. Spread in an even layer on a rimmed baking sheet.

3. Bake until the fennel begins to brown, about 40 minutes, flipping after about 20 minutes.

4. Toss with the lemon zest before serving.

FLAVOR BOOST: Instead of lemon zest, toss with ¼ cup of grated Parmesan cheese.

PER SERVING: *Calories: 96; Total fat: 7g; Sodium: 352mg; Carbohydrates: 9g; Fiber: 4g; Protein: 2g*

Honey works well to soothe acid reflux—unless you're sensitive to FODMAPs, in which case you'll want to avoid it (see the Substitution Tip). The sweetness of the honey is a good match for the earthy, caramelized flavors of the carrots.

HONEY-ROASTED CARROTS

SERVES: 4 · **PREP TIME:** 10 minutes · **COOK TIME:** 40 minutes

GLUTEN-FREE

VEGETARIAN

*2 cups baby carrots,
  halved lengthwise*
2 tablespoons olive oil
¼ cup honey
½ teaspoon sea salt

1. Preheat the oven to 400°F.

2. In a large bowl, toss the carrots with the olive oil, honey, and salt. Place in a single layer on a baking sheet.

3. Bake until the carrots soften and begin to brown, about 40 minutes, flipping after about 20 minutes.

SUBSTITUTION TIP: Make this low-FODMAP by replacing the honey with an equal amount of pure maple syrup.

PER SERVING: *Calories: 142; Total fat: 7g; Sodium: 322mg; Carbohydrates: 22g; Fiber: 1g; Protein: 1g*

Yogurt, rather than the traditional butter or shortening, makes these biscuits tender. Be sure to choose nonfat plain yogurt and not Greek yogurt, which has too much protein. These biscuits are a delicious side dish, or make a breakfast sandwich with the Sage-Turkey Breakfast Sausage (page 27) or use them as a base for strawberry shortcake.

NO-FAT BISCUITS

SERVES: 6 • **PREP TIME:** 10 minutes • **COOK TIME:** 25 minutes

VEGETARIAN

Nonstick cooking spray
2 cups all-purpose flour
¾ teaspoon baking soda
2 teaspoons baking powder
Pinch sea salt
1¼ cups nonfat plain yogurt

1. Preheat the oven to 425°F. Spray a rimmed baking sheet with nonstick cooking spray.

2. In a medium bowl, whisk together the flour, baking soda, baking powder, and salt.

3. Fold in the yogurt until just mixed.

4. Use a large spoon to form 6 biscuits on the prepared baking sheet.

5. Bake until the biscuits are golden brown, 20 to 25 minutes.

BATCH IT: These biscuits will freeze well, so feel free to make a double or triple batch and freeze them in zip-top bags for up to 6 months.

PER SERVING: Calories: 161; Total fat: 0g; Sodium: 373mg; Carbohydrates: 34g; Fiber: 1g; Protein: 7g

This crumbly, moist cornbread is delicious with a little honey drizzled on it, or it's good with soups and stews as a side dish. You can use the recipe to make cornbread pancakes by cooking them in a hot non-stick skillet with a little bit of nonstick cooking spray or oil. It's a versatile recipe you can use for all kinds of meals.

EASY CORNBREAD

SERVES: 6 • **PREP TIME:** 10 minutes • **COOK TIME:** 20 minutes

VEGETARIAN

Nonstick cooking spray
¾ cup all-purpose flour
1½ cups cornmeal
1 tablespoon baking powder
¼ teaspoon sea salt
1 large egg, beaten
1 cup nonfat milk

1. Preheat the oven to 425°F. Spray a 9-inch baking pan with nonstick cooking spray.

2. In a medium bowl, whisk together the flour, cornmeal, baking powder, and salt.

3. In a small bowl, whisk together the egg and milk.

4. Add the wet ingredients to the dry and fold together until just combined. Pour into the prepared pan.

5. Bake until browned, about 20 minutes.

FLAVOR BOOST: Mix in ½ cup of grated Monterey Jack cheese before baking to add a cheesy flavor to the cornbread, or stir up to 1 teaspoon of grated orange zest into the dry ingredients.

PER SERVING: Calories: 188; Total fat: 2g; Sodium: 380mg; Carbohydrates: 37g; Fiber: 3g; Protein: 6g

Shredding Brussels sprouts on a box grater or cutting them into thin strips with a sharp knife helps them cook quickly. And with their alkalinity, Brussels sprouts are great for GERD and other digestive issues. Jazz up this basic recipe by adding your favorite GERD-friendly ground spices or herbs.

SHREDDED BRUSSELS SPROUTS

SERVES: 4 · **PREP TIME:** 10 minutes · **COOK TIME:** 7 minutes

GLUTEN-FREE

VEGAN

1 tablespoon olive oil

8 ounces Brussels sprouts, shredded or julienned

½ teaspoon sea salt

Place a large nonstick skillet over medium-high heat and add the olive oil. Once the oil is shimmering, add the Brussels sprouts and salt. Cook, stirring occasionally, until the sprouts are browned, 5 to 7 minutes.

FLAVOR BOOST: Toss with ¼ cup grated reduced-fat Parmesan cheese before serving.

PER SERVING: *Calories: 54; Total fat: 4g; Sodium: 305mg; Carbohydrates: 5g; Fiber: 2g; Protein: 2g*

While these beets take about an hour to cook, most of it is inactive time, so they're still easy to make. Maple and ginger complement the sweet, earthy flavor of the beets, and the ginger can quickly soothe GERD and acid reflux, so it's a great ingredient to add.

MAPLE-GINGER ROASTED BEETS

SERVES: 4 · **PREP TIME:** 10 minutes · **COOK TIME:** 1 hour

GLUTEN-FREE
VEGAN

8 ounces beets, peeled and quartered
2 tablespoons olive oil
½ teaspoon sea salt
1 tablespoon grated fresh ginger
¼ cup pure maple syrup

1. Preheat the oven to 400°F.

2. Place the beets on a rimmed baking sheet and drizzle with the olive oil. Toss to coat. Sprinkle with the salt and ginger.

3. Roast for 30 minutes. Remove from the oven. Drizzle the beets with the syrup and stir to mix. Return to the oven and continue roasting for 30 minutes more.

SUBSTITUTION TIP: To make this low-FODMAP, replace the beets with an equal amount of carrots or parsnips.

PER SERVING: Calories: 137; Total fat: 7g; Sodium: 337mg; Carbohydrates: 19g; Fiber: 2g; Protein: 1g

Kale is a great food for acid reflux because of its alkalinity, and it's low in FODMAPs and high in nutrition. These crispy baked kale chips are also low in fat, but they don't sacrifice on flavor because they're dusted with a mix of ginger and cumin. They're delicious on their own or with in a nonfat yogurt–based dip.

GINGER-CUMIN KALE CHIPS

SERVES: 6 · **PREP TIME:** 10 minutes · **COOK TIME:** 20 minutes

GLUTEN-FREE
LOW-FODMAP
VEGAN

1 bunch kale, stems removed and leaves trimmed
1 tablespoon olive oil
½ teaspoon sea salt
1 tablespoon grated fresh ginger
½ teaspoon ground cumin

1. Preheat the oven to 350°F. Line a rimmed baking sheet with parchment paper.

2. In a large bowl, toss the kale leaves with the olive oil, salt, ginger, and cumin.

3. Spread in an even layer on the prepared baking pan.

4. Bake until the kale is crisp and starting to brown, about 20 minutes, flipping after about 10 minutes.

INGREDIENT TIP: Wash the kale thoroughly and spin it dry in a salad spinner or let it drip dry in a colander. Then pat each leaf dry before you use it to ensure that the kale will crisp in the oven.

PER SERVING: *Calories: 40; Total fat: 3g; Sodium: 209mg; Carbohydrates: 4g; Fiber: 1g; Protein: 1g*

These mashed sweet potatoes are loaded with sweet, earthy flavor combined with the slight bite of acid reflux–soothing ginger. The ginger and sweet potatoes are not overly sweet, so they make a delicious side dish for fish, poultry, or meat. Alternatively, top them with Mushroom and Fennel Stew (page 67) for a delicious vegetarian meal.

GINGER MASHED SWEET POTATOES

SERVES: 4 · **PREP TIME:** 10 minutes · **COOK TIME:** 20 minutes

GLUTEN-FREE
VEGETARIAN

2 sweet potatoes, peeled and cut into 1-inch pieces
1 tablespoon grated fresh ginger
½ cup nonfat milk or nondairy milk
¼ cup nonfat plain yogurt
½ teaspoon sea salt

1. Place the sweet potatoes in a large pot and cover with at least 2 inches of water. Place over medium-high heat and bring to a boil.

2. Cover and cook until the potatoes are tender, about 15 minutes.

3. Drain the potatoes and return them to the pot. Add the ginger, milk, yogurt, and salt.

4. Mash with a potato masher until smooth, and then stir well to combine.

SUBSTITUTION TIP: You can make this lower in FODMAPs by replacing the sweet potatoes with 3 cups of butternut squash cubes.

PER SERVING: *Calories: 87; Total fat: <1g; Sodium: 322mg; Carbohydrates: 19g; Fiber: 2g; Protein: 3g*

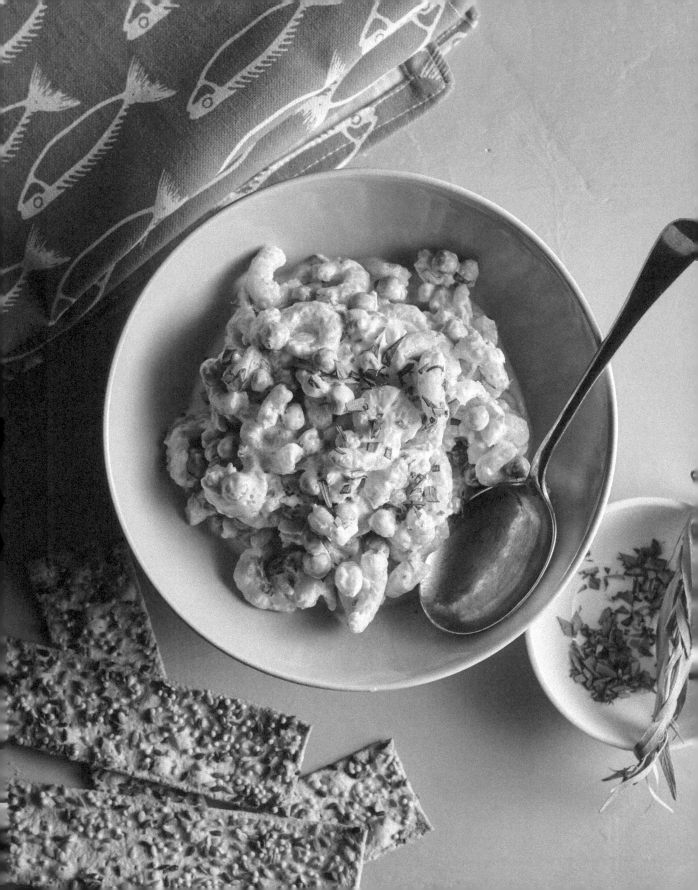

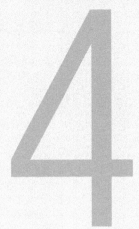

Soups and Salads

Melon is highly alkaline and cooling, making it the ideal ingredient for fighting acid reflux. This salad is simple, and will keep for a few days in the refrigerator, so it makes a wonderful side dish, dessert, or snack. If you'd like a slightly heartier snack, add up to ½ cup of nonfat plain yogurt and a few tablespoons of honey or pure maple syrup. If you're sensitive to FODMAPs, don't consume more than about ½ cup of melon at a time.

SIMPLE MELON BALL SALAD

SERVES: 4 • **PREP TIME:** 10 minutes

GLUTEN-FREE
VEGAN

2 cups assorted melon balls
1 tablespoon grated fresh ginger

In a large bowl, combine the melon balls and ginger. Mix well.

INGREDIENT TIP: Use a melon ball scoop to create the balls, or chop the melons with a knife into cubes. Be sure to remove the seeds. If you're sensitive to FODMAPs, avoid watermelon and use cantaloupe, honeydew, or casaba melon or a combination.

PER SERVING: *Calories: 33; Total fat: <1g; Sodium: 16mg; Carbohydrates: 8g; Fiber: 1g; Protein: 1g*

Carrots are soothing for acid reflux, so this flavorful salad makes a perfect GERD-friendly meal. Grate carrots on a box grater for the perfect texture. This salad will keep well for up to 3 days in the refrigerator, but it doesn't freeze well, so eat it within a few days.

SHREDDED CARROT AND GINGER SALAD

SERVES: 4 · **PREP TIME:** 10 minutes

GLUTEN-FREE
VEGETARIAN

¼ **cup nonfat plain yogurt**
1 **tablespoon grated fresh ginger**
1 **tablespoon pure maple syrup**
6 **carrots, grated**

1. In a medium bowl, whisk together the yogurt, ginger, and syrup.

2. Add the grated carrots and mix well.

FLAVOR BOOST: Add ¼ cup of raisins and 2 tablespoons of pepitas (hulled pumpkin seeds) to add extra flavor and crunch.

PER SERVING: *Calories: 58; Total fat: <1g; Sodium: 74mg; Carbohydrates: 13g; Fiber: 3g; Protein: 2g*

Fennel has a lovely anise flavor, and it's a highly alka-line root vegetable that's soothing for GERD. It also has a nice celery-like crunch. Be sure to use red apples, which are far more GERD-friendly than green apples. A simple maple-yogurt dressing adds sweet-ness to this yummy salad.

SHAVED FENNEL AND RED APPLE SALAD

SERVES: 4 · **PREP TIME:** 10 minutes

GLUTEN-FREE
VEGETARIAN

¼ cup nonfat plain yogurt
1 tablespoon grated
  fresh ginger
1 tablespoon pure
  maple syrup
1 fennel bulb, julienned or
  grated on a box grater
2 red apples, peeled, cored,
  and julienned or grated
  on a box grater

1. In a medium bowl, whisk together the yogurt, ginger, and syrup.

2. Add the fennel and apple and mix well.

SUBSTITUTION TIP: To make this low-FODMAP, replace the apples with 1 jicama root, peeled and julienned, and limit each serving to ½ cup. Replace the yogurt with a nonfat, nondairy plain yogurt.

PER SERVING: Calories: 75; Total fat: <1g; Sodium: 41mg; Carbohydrates: 18g; Fiber: 4g; Protein: 2g

Egg salad is easy and delicious, whether you serve it as a salad or put it in a pita and have a sandwich. This version has GERD-soothing fennel added for crunch and flavor. You can make it ahead and it will keep for up to 3 days in the refrigerator.

CRUNCHY EGG SALAD

SERVES: 4 · **PREP TIME:** 10 minutes

GLUTEN-FREE
VEGETARIAN

¼ *cup nonfat plain yogurt*
1 *tablespoon chopped fennel fronds*
½ *teaspoon sea salt*
6 *large hardboiled eggs, peeled and chopped*
½ *fennel bulb, minced*

1. In a medium bowl, whisk together the yogurt, fennel fronds, and salt.

2. Add the eggs and fennel. Mix well.

FLAVOR BOOST: Mix 2 teaspoons of Dijon mustard into the yogurt to add flavor to the dressing.

PER SERVING: Calories: 133; Total fat: 8g; Sodium: 409mg; Carbohydrates: 4g; Fiber: 1g; Protein: 11g

You can buy precooked baby shrimp in the seafood department at the grocery store, so it's the perfect ingredient for this quick and easy seafood salad. Fresh or thawed frozen peas add texture along with a sweet, earthy flavor. The peas also have an alkaline effect that can help calm GERD.

SIMPLE SHRIMP SALAD

SERVES: 4 · **PREP TIME:** 10 minutes

GLUTEN-FREE

¼ cup nonfat plain yogurt

2 tablespoons chopped fresh tarragon

½ teaspoon sea salt

8 ounces cooked baby shrimp, rinsed and drained

½ cup fresh or frozen peas, thawed

1. In a medium bowl, whisk together the yogurt, tarragon, and salt.

2. Add the shrimp and peas. Mix well.

SUBSTITUTION TIP: Make this low-FODMAP by replacing the peas with ½ cup of chopped fresh fennel or 1 stalk of chopped celery.

PER SERVING: *Calories: 79; Total fat: 1g; Sodium: 448mg; Carbohydrates: 4g; Fiber: 1g; Protein: 14g*

This cooling soup is the perfect summer snack or lunch. Easy and quick, it's best if you chill it before serving. You can substitute honeydew or casaba melon for the cantaloupe if you prefer a slightly different flavor profile. Use watermelon with caution either due to FODMAPs or if you've noticed that watermelon seems to trigger acid reflux for you.

CHILLED GINGER-MELON SOUP

SERVES: 4 · **PREP TIME:** 10 minutes, plus chilling time

GLUTEN-FREE
VEGETARIAN

6 cups cantaloupe cubes
½ cup skim milk or
nondairy milk
1 tablespoon honey
1 tablespoon grated
fresh ginger
½ teaspoon grated lime zest
Pinch sea salt

1. In a blender or food processor, combine all the ingredients. Blend until smooth.

2. Chill for 2 hours. Blend again before serving.

SUBSTITUTION TIP: To make this low-FODMAP, replace the honey with a packet of stevia or omit the sweetener altogether.

PER SERVING: Calories: 112; Total fat: 1g; Sodium: 54mg; Carbohydrates: 26g; Fiber: 2g; Protein: 3g

Buying cooked rotisserie chicken is the perfect time-saver for this simple and tasty soup. Remove the skin and bones from the white meat and shred the breast before adding it to your soup. You can freeze the rest of the chicken meat in single servings in zip-top bags for up to 6 months and use the carcass to make Homemade Chicken Broth (page 116).

CHICKEN NOODLE SOUP

SERVES: 4 · **PREP TIME:** 10 minutes · **COOK TIME:** 15 minutes

1 tablespoon olive oil
1 fennel bulb, chopped
5 cups chicken broth, store-bought or Homemade Chicken Broth
3 cups shredded cooked chicken breast
½ teaspoon sea salt
4 ounces whole-wheat spaghetti noodles

1. Place a large pot over medium-high heat and add the olive oil. Once the oil shimmers, add the fennel and cook, stirring occasionally, until browned, about 5 minutes.

2. Add the chicken broth, shredded chicken, and salt. Bring to a boil.

3. Add the spaghetti and bring back to a boil. Cook until the noodles are tender, 8 to 12 minutes.

SUBSTITUTION TIP: Make this gluten-free and low-FODMAP by replacing the spaghetti with zucchini noodles. (You can find them in the produce section of your grocery store or make them yourself using a spiralizer or vegetable peeler.) Reduce the cooking time to 5 minutes after adding the zucchini noodles.

PER SERVING: Calories: 373; Total fat: 14g; Sodium: 411mg; Carbohydrates: 29g; Fiber: 5g; Protein: 36g

You can make cream of any vegetable soup by following this simple recipe and replacing the asparagus with an equal amount of another vegetable such as broccoli or cauliflower. The alkalinity of the vegetables is good for GERD, and if you're FODMAP sensitive, you can replace the asparagus with a lower-FODMAP veggie.

CREAM OF ASPARAGUS SOUP

SERVES: 4 • **PREP TIME:** 10 minutes • **COOK TIME:** 15 minutes

GLUTEN-FREE
VEGETARIAN

1 tablespoon olive oil
2 bunches asparagus, trimmed and chopped
5 cups vegetable broth, store-bought or Home-made Vegetable Broth (page 114)
½ teaspoon sea salt
1 cup nonfat plain yogurt
2 tablespoons chopped fresh dill

1. Place a large pot over medium-high heat and add the olive oil. When the oil shimmers, add the asparagus and cook, stirring occasionally for 5 minutes.

2. Add the vegetable broth and salt. Bring to a simmer. Cover and cook until the asparagus is tender, about 5 minutes.

3. Remove the pot from the heat. Stir in the yogurt. Transfer the soup to a blender or food processor and blend until smooth.

4. Stir in the dill.

INGREDIENT TIP: To trim the asparagus, hold each stalk about 1 inch from either end and bend. The asparagus will break at the top of the woody, tough part. Discard the tough stems and keep the tender stalks.

PER SERVING: *Calories: 119; Total fat: 4g; Sodium: 347mg; Carbohydrates: 17g; Fiber: 5g; Protein: 9g*

Save prep time with this recipe by purchasing pre-cut butternut squash or using frozen cubed butternut squash in place of the fresh. When using pre-cut squash, use about 3 cups. This soup freezes well, so you can double or triple the batch and keep it in single-serving airtight containers in the freezer. Reheat in the microwave.

BUTTERNUT SQUASH SOUP

SERVES: 4 · **PREP TIME:** 10 minutes · **COOK TIME:** 15 minutes

GLUTEN-FREE
VEGETARIAN

1 butternut squash, peeled, seeded, and cut into cubes
5 cups vegetable broth, store-bought or Homemade Vegetable Broth (page 114)
1 teaspoon ground cumin
1 teaspoon grated fresh ginger
½ teaspoon sea salt
1 cup plain nonfat yogurt

1. Place the butternut squash, vegetable broth, cumin, ginger, and salt in a large pot over medium-high heat. Bring to a boil and boil until the squash is tender, about 10 minutes.

2. Transfer the soup to a blender or food processor. Add the yogurt and puree until smooth.

FLAVOR BOOST: Garnish the soup with 2 tablespoons of pepitas (pumpkin seeds) for a delicious crunchy upgrade.

PER SERVING: *Calories: 101; Total fat: <1g; Sodium: 350mg; Carbohydrates: 23g; Fiber: 5g; Protein: 5g*

Using dried porcini mushrooms boosts the mushroom flavor of this soup significantly, so you wind up with an earthy, flavorful soup. You can boost flavor even more by stirring in chopped, fresh thyme to the cooked soup, which perfectly complements the earthy flavors of the mushrooms.

GOLDEN MUSHROOM SOUP

SERVES: 4 · **PREP TIME:** 10 minutes · **COOK TIME:** 15 minutes

GLUTEN-FREE
VEGAN

2 ounces dried porcini mushrooms
6 cups vegetable broth, store-bought or Homemade Vegetable Broth (page 114), boiling
1 tablespoon olive oil
8 ounces sliced mushrooms
1 teaspoon dried thyme
½ teaspoon sea salt

1. In a large heatproof bowl, soak the porcini mushrooms in the hot vegetable broth until soft, 30 minutes. Strain the broth from the porcini mushrooms, reserving both, and chop the porcini mushrooms into small pieces.

2. Place a large pot over medium-high heat and add the olive oil. When it shimmers, add the sliced mushrooms, thyme, and salt. Cook, stirring occasionally, until the mushrooms brown, about 7 minutes.

3. Add the reserved broth and chopped porcini mushrooms to the pot. Bring to a simmer. Cook, stirring occasionally, for 5 minutes.

BATCH IT: This freezes exceptionally well. Make a double or triple batch to freeze in single-serving airtight containers for meals on the go.

PER SERVING: Calories: 108; Total fat: 4g; Sodium: 307mg; Carbohydrates: 12g; Fiber: 4g; Protein: 6g

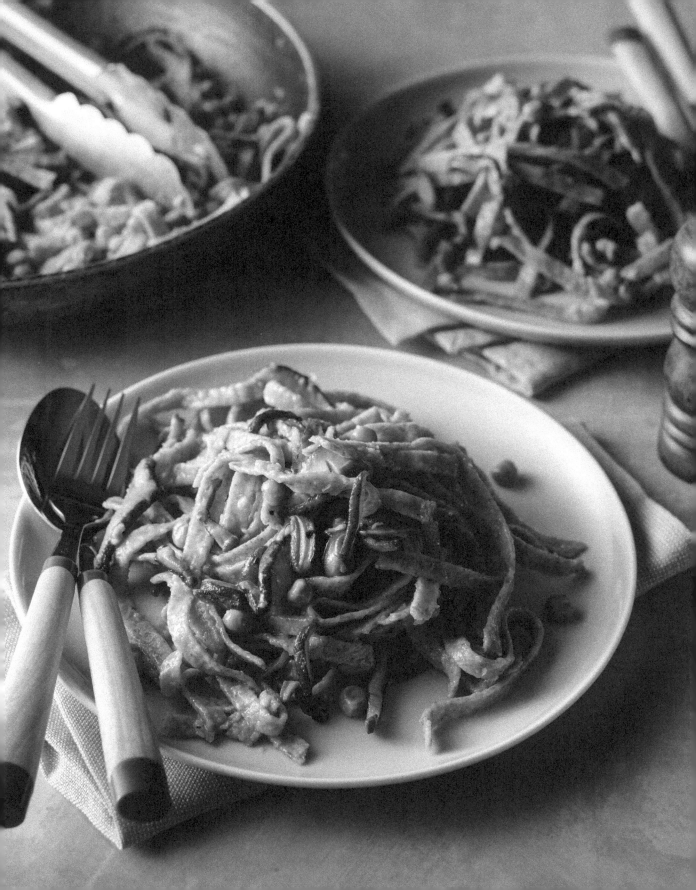

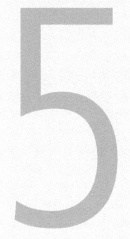

Vegetarian and Vegan Mains

This is a simple but delicious quick pasta recipe that uses acid reflux–soothing ginger. If you'd like to add a little texture, add a tablespoon of chopped peanuts or opt for a crunchy peanut butter. You can also add a few dashes of sesame oil to the sauce for additional flavor, but don't add much more than about ½ teaspoon to keep added fat to a minimum.

PEANUT BUTTER NOODLES

SERVES: 4 · **PREP TIME:** 10 minutes · **COOK TIME:** 10 minutes

VEGAN

¼ *cup peanut butter*

1 tablespoon low-sodium soy sauce

¼ *cup vegetable broth, store-bought or Homemade Vegetable Broth (page 114)*

1 tablespoon grated fresh ginger

8 ounces whole-wheat spaghetti, cooked according to package instructions and drained

1. In a blender or food processor, combine the peanut butter, soy sauce, vegetable broth, and ginger. Blend well.

2. Place the hot noodles in a large bowl. Pour the sauce over and toss with the noodles.

SUBSTITUTION TIP: To make this recipe low-FODMAP and gluten-free, replace the soy sauce with tamari and replace the whole-wheat noodles with gluten-free noodles.

PER SERVING: Calories: 279; Total fat: 10g; Sodium: 251mg; Carbohydrates: 45g; Fiber: 7g; Protein: 10g

Make this easy tofu stir-fry as a topping for steamed rice to create a full, filling meal. You can add fresh flavors to the stir-fry by including extra veggies such as broccoli florets or fresh peas, and if you enjoy cilantro, garnish the finished dish with a few tablespoons of chopped fresh cilantro.

GINGER TOFU STIR-FRY

SERVES: 4 · **PREP TIME:** 10 minutes · **COOK TIME:** 5 minutes

VEGAN

1 tablespoon oil

8 ounces extra-firm tofu, cut into pieces

8 ounces shiitake mushrooms, sliced

2 tablespoons grated fresh ginger

1 tablespoon low-sodium soy sauce or tamari

1. Place a large nonstick skillet over medium-high heat and add the oil. Once the oil shimmers, add the tofu, mushrooms, and ginger. Cook, stirring constantly, until the mushrooms are tender and the tofu cooked, about 5 minutes.

2. Add the soy sauce. Cook, stirring constantly, for 1 minute more.

SUBSTITUTION TIP: To make this recipe FODMAP-friendly, omit the tofu and shiitake mushrooms and instead use 1 pound of oyster mushrooms, which are low in polyols.

PER SERVING: *Calories: 119; Total fat: 6g; Sodium: 163mg; Carbohydrates: 11g; Fiber: 2g; Protein: 7g*

This makes a delicious main dish or a yummy break-fast side dish. The ginger both flavors the hash and helps reduce GERD, while the alkalinity of the potato and kale is also beneficial for people struggling with acid reflux.

KALE AND SWEET POTATO HASH

SERVES: 4 • **PREP TIME:** 10 minutes • **COOK TIME:** 10 minutes

VEGAN

2 tablespoons oil

2 sweet potatoes, peeled and cut into ½-inch pieces

1 bunch kale, stems removed and leaves chopped

1 teaspoon grated fresh ginger

½ teaspoon ground cumin

½ teaspoon sea salt

1. Place a large nonstick skillet over medium-high heat and add the oil. Once the oil shimmers, add the potatoes, kale, ginger, cumin, and salt.

2. Cook, stirring occasionally, until the potatoes soften and begin to brown, 10 to 15 minutes.

SUBSTITUTION TIP: To make this recipe FODMAP-friendly, replace the sweet potatoes with 2 cups of peeled and chopped carrots.

PER SERVING: *Calories: 157; Total fat: 8g; Sodium: 322mg; Carbohydrates: 22g; Fiber: 4g; Protein: 3g*

Portobello mushrooms make great burgers, and they're super easy to grill in a grill pan, outdoors, or even on an indoor grill such as a countertop grill if you have one. Prepare the mushrooms by using a spoon to scrape the black gills from the underside of the mushrooms after you remove the stems. You can save the stems in a zip-top bag in the freezer to make Homemade Vegetable Broth (page 114) but discard the gills.

GRILLED PORTOBELLO MUSHROOM BURGER

SERVES: 4 • **PREP TIME:** 10 minutes • **COOK TIME:** 10 minutes

VEGAN

1 tablespoon olive oil

1 tablespoon low-sodium soy sauce

4 portobello mushrooms, stems and gills removed

½ avocado, peeled, pitted, and sliced

4 whole-wheat hamburger buns, toasted

1. Preheat a grill or grill pan on high heat.

2. In a small bowl, whisk together the olive oil and soy sauce. Brush on both sides of the mushroom caps.

3. Grill until soft, about 5 minutes per side.

4. Mash the avocado and spread on the toasted buns. Top with the mushrooms.

INGREDIENT TIP: You can also roast the mushrooms in the oven. Brush with the oil and soy sauce and then roast in a preheated 400°F oven for about 30 minutes, flipping halfway through.

PER SERVING: *Calories: 221; Total fat: 9g; Sodium: 341mg; Carbohydrates: 31g; Fiber: 7g; Protein: 9g*

This stew is flavored with fennel, which has a lovely anise flavor and a nice crunch. It also is soothing for acid reflux, so it's a great ingredient to include in acid reflux recipes. You can make a gluten-free stew by substituting any other flour—such as rice flour—for the all-purpose flour.

CHICKPEA AND FENNEL STEW

SERVES: 4 · **PREP TIME:** 10 minutes · **COOK TIME:** 10 minutes

VEGAN

2 tablespoons oil
1 fennel bulb, chopped
2 tablespoons
*   all-purpose flour*
3 cups vegetable broth,
*   store-bought or*
*   Homemade Vegetable*
*   Broth (page 114)*
2 (14-ounce) cans
*   chickpeas, drained*
½ teaspoon sea salt
2 tablespoons chopped
*   fennel fronds*

1. Place a large pot over medium-high heat and add the oil. Once the oil shimmers, add the fennel bulb and cook, stirring occasionally, until the fennel starts to soften, about 4 minutes.

2. Add the flour and cook, stirring constantly, for 1 minute.

3. Add the vegetable broth. Use the side of the spoon to scrape any browned bits from the bottom of the pot.

4. Add the chickpeas and salt. Bring to a simmer, and then reduce the heat to maintain that simmer. Cook, stirring frequently, until the chickpeas are heated through and the sauce thickens, about 5 minutes.

5. Remove the pot from the heat and stir in the fennel fronds.

FLAVOR BOOST: Add the grated zest of half an orange when you add the broth for additional flavoring.

PER SERVING: *Calories: 307; Total fat: 9g; Sodium: 574mg; Carbohydrates: 47g; Fiber: 13g; Protein: 12g*

This risotto comes together easily because instead of you standing over a hot stove stirring and stirring and stirring, the magic happens while the rice is in the oven.

OVEN-BAKED PEA AND PORCINI RISOTTO

SERVES: 6 · **PREP TIME:** 10 minutes · **COOK TIME:** 45 minutes

GLUTEN-FREE
VEGAN

2 ounces dried porcini mushrooms
5 cups vegetable broth, store-bought or Homemade Vegetable Broth (page 114)
1½ cups Arborio rice
1 cup fresh or frozen peas
1 teaspoon dried thyme
½ teaspoon sea salt

1. Preheat the oven to 350°F.

2. In a large pan, combine the dried mushrooms and broth. Place over high heat and bring to a boil. Reduce the heat to low and simmer for 5 minutes.

3. Remove the pan from the heat. Strain the broth from the mushrooms, reserving both. Chop the mushrooms.

4. In a covered casserole dish or large ovenproof pot, combine the chopped mushrooms, reserved vegetable broth, rice, peas, thyme, and salt. Stir to combine.

5. Cover and cook in the oven until the liquid is absorbed and the rice tender, 40 to 45 minutes.

6. Stir before serving.

FLAVOR BOOST: Stir in ½ cup of grated Parmesan cheese when the risotto comes out of the oven.

PER SERVING: Calories: 221; Total fat: <1g; Sodium: 228mg; Carbohydrates: 46g; Fiber: 4g; Protein: 7g

Pasta carbonara is typically made with bacon and eggs. In this case, thinly sliced shiitake mushrooms stand in for the bacon, adding a nice crisp texture and umami flavor. Peas are an alkaline legume that can also help soothe acid reflux while adding color to the finished dish. If you're worried about the texture of the eggs or the heat from the pasta scrambling the eggs as you add them, whisk them with up to 2 tablespoons of nondairy milk before adding to the hot pasta.

MUSHROOM PASTA CARBONARA

SERVES: 4 · **PREP TIME:** 10 minutes · **COOK TIME:** 10 minutes

---

VEGETARIAN

2 tablespoons olive oil

4 ounces shiitake mushrooms, stems removed and caps thinly sliced

8 ounces whole-wheat spaghetti, cooked according to package instructions and drained

1 cup fresh or frozen peas

4 large eggs, beaten

½ teaspoon sea salt

1. Place a large nonstick skillet over medium-high heat and add the olive oil. Once the oil shimmers, add the mushrooms in a single layer and cook, without stirring, until they begin to brown on one side, about 5 minutes. Stir and cook for 3 to 4 minutes more until they are golden and crisped.

2. Add the spaghetti and peas. Cook until the peas are warmed through, about 2 minutes.

3. In a small bowl, whisk the eggs with the salt.

4. Remove the pan from the heat. Pour the eggs in a thin stream into the pasta, stirring as you do. The residual heat from the pasta will cook the eggs just enough to make a sauce.

_____

SUBSTITUTION TIP: If you're sensitive to gluten, you can replace the spaghetti with zucchini noodles or gluten-free pasta.

_____

PER SERVING: *Calories: 355; Total fat: 14g; Sodium: 403mg; Carbohydrates: 50g; Fiber: 8g; Protein: 15g*

This simple casserole keeps very well in the freezer, so you can cut it into single servings and freeze in zip-top bags for up to 6 months. Simply thaw and reheat in the microwave. The fennel adds crunch, and both the zucchini and fennel are alkaline and can help soothe acid reflux while adding flavor and texture.

FENNEL, ZUCCHINI, AND EGG CASSEROLE

SERVES: 4 · **PREP TIME:** 10 minutes · **COOK TIME:** 45 minutes

GLUTEN-FREE
VEGETARIAN

Nonstick cooking spray
1 medium zucchini, grated
1 fennel bulb, grated
8 large eggs, beaten
½ cup skim milk
½ teaspoon sea salt
½ cup grated fat-free Cheddar cheese

1. Preheat the oven to 350°F. Spray a 9-inch square baking dish with nonstick cooking spray.

2. Evenly layer the zucchini and fennel in the bottom of the dish.

3. In a large bowl, whisk together the eggs, milk, and salt. Fold in the cheese. Pour the egg mixture over the vegetables.

4. Bake, uncovered, until the eggs are set, about 45 minutes.

BATCH IT: This freezes well. Double the batch and cook in a 9-by-13-inch baking dish for about 65 minutes, or until the eggs set.

PER SERVING: Calories: 203; Total fat: 10g; Sodium: 636mg; Carbohydrates: 9g; Fiber: 2g; Protein: 19g

Both kale and white beans are deliciously alkaline, so they're perfect for people struggling with acid reflux. You can make this gluten-free if you're sensitive by replacing the all-purpose flour with any gluten-free flour, which will still give the stew a satisfying and thick texture.

WHITE BEAN AND KALE STEW

SERVES: 4 · **PREP TIME:** 10 minutes · **COOK TIME:** 10 minutes

VEGAN

2 tablespoons olive oil

1 bunch kale, stems removed and leaves chopped

2 tablespoons all-purpose flour

3 cups vegetable broth, store-bought or Homemade Vegetable Broth (page 114)

2 (14-ounce) cans white beans, drained

½ teaspoon sea salt

1. Place a large pot over medium-high heat and add the oil. Once the oil shimmers, add the kale and cook, stirring occasionally, until it begins to soften, about 5 minutes.

2. Add the flour and cook, stirring constantly, for 1 minute.

3. Add the broth, beans, and salt. Bring to a simmer. Cook, stirring frequently, until the sauce thickens, about 5 minutes.

FLAVOR BOOST: Make a gremolata to stir into the finished stew by mixing together ¼ cup of chopped Italian parsley and 1 tablespoon grated orange zest. Stir into the stew just before serving.

PER SERVING: *Calories: 263; Total fat: 7g; Sodium: 792mg; Carbohydrates: 43g; Fiber: 13g; Protein: 15g*

While many people think couscous is a grain like rice, it's actually tiny bits of pasta, so it cooks very quickly. With alkaline carrots, this colorful dish is GERD-friendly, with lots of flavor. It will keep in the refrigerator in an airtight container for up to 5 days.

LENTIL AND VEGGIE COUSCOUS

SERVES: 4 · **PREP TIME:** 10 minutes · **COOK TIME:** 10 minutes

GLUTEN-FREE
VEGAN

2 tablespoons olive oil
2 carrots, chopped
2 cups vegetable broth, store-bought or Homemade Vegetable Broth (page 114)
1 cup instant couscous
2 (14-ounce) cans lentils
½ teaspoon sea salt

1. Place a medium pot over medium-high heat and add the oil. Once the oil shimmers, add the carrots and cook, stirring occasionally, until the carrots begin to soften, about 5 minutes.

2. Add the broth and bring to a boil.

3. Add the couscous. Cover the pot and remove it from the heat. Let sit, covered, for 10 minutes.

4. Meanwhile, place the lentils in another medium pot. Cook over medium heat, stirring occasionally, until warmed through, about 5 minutes. Drain.

5. Fluff the couscous with a fork. Stir in the hot lentils and salt.

FLAVOR BOOST: Add up to ¼ of a red bell pepper, ribs and seeds removed and finely chopped. Combine with the couscous when you add the lentils for a boost of flavor, texture, and color.

PER SERVING: Calories: 438; Total fat: 8g; Sodium: 740mg; Carbohydrates: 72g; Fiber: 16g; Protein: 22g

You can find cooked rice in the rice aisle of the grocery store or cook a large batch yourself and freeze it in 1-cup servings in zip-top bags for up to 6 months. You can also substitute riced cauliflower (available in the freezer section at the grocery) in place of the cooked rice if you prefer.

FRIED RICE

SERVES: 4 • **PREP TIME:** 5 minutes • **COOK TIME:** 10 minutes

VEGAN

2 tablespoons olive oil
2 cups fresh or frozen peas
2 tablespoons grated
*   fresh ginger*
2 cups cooked brown rice
1 tablespoon low-sodium
*   soy sauce*

1. Place a large nonstick skillet over medium-high heat and add the oil. Once the oil shimmers, add the peas, ginger, and rice. Cook, stirring frequently, until the rice and peas are warmed through, about 5 minutes.

2. Add the soy sauce. Cook, stirring, for 1 minute more.

SUBSTITUTION TIP: Make this low-FODMAP by replacing the peas with 2 chopped carrots. Cook the carrots for about 4 minutes in the oil to soften them before adding the ginger and the rice.

PER SERVING: *Calories: 229; Total fat: 8g; Sodium: 226mg; Carbohydrates: 33g; Fiber: 5g; Protein: 6g*

With alkaline fennel and mushrooms, this stew is the perfect GERD-friendly meal. It's also loaded with delicious, savory flavors that make it warming and hearty, perfect for a fall or winter meal when you're looking for something to stick to your ribs.

MUSHROOM AND FENNEL STEW

SERVES: 4 · **PREP TIME:** 10 minutes · **COOK TIME:** 10 minutes

VEGAN

2 tablespoons olive oil

1 pound cremini mushrooms, stems removed and caps chopped

1 fennel bulb, finely chopped

½ teaspoon sea salt

2 tablespoons all-purpose flour

3 cups vegetable, store-bought or Homemade Vegetable Broth (page 114)

1. Place a large nonstick skillet over medium-high heat and add the olive oil. Once the oil shimmers, add the mushrooms, fennel, and salt. Cook, stirring occasionally, until the fennel is soft, about 5 minutes.

2. Add the flour and cook, stirring constantly, for 1 minute.

3. Add the vegetable broth. Bring to a simmer while stirring. Cook, stirring, until the broth thickens, about 5 minutes.

FLAVOR BOOST: Stir in up to ¼ cup of grated Parmesan cheese just before serving.

PER SERVING: *Calories: 122; Total fat: 8g; Sodium: 332mg; Carbohydrates: 12g; Fiber: 3g; Protein: 5g*

Slice the eggplant very thin to make this super tasty. You can do this in a food processor, using a mandoline, or using a very sharp and steady knife. Try for ⅛-inch-thick eggplant slices for best results. You can also use any vegan cream cheese in place of the nonfat cream cheese, provided you know it doesn't aggravate your GERD.

BAKED MUSHROOM-STUFFED EGGPLANT ROLLS

SERVES: 4 · **PREP TIME:** 10 minutes · **COOK TIME:** 55 minutes

VEGETARIAN

2 tablespoons olive oil
8 ounces mushrooms, finely chopped
½ teaspoon sea salt
1 teaspoon dried thyme
4 ounces fat-free cream cheese, cut into pieces
1 eggplant, very thinly sliced lengthwise

1. Preheat the oven to 350°F. Line a 9-inch baking dish with parchment paper.

2. Place a large nonstick skillet over medium-high heat and add the olive oil. Once the oil shimmers, add the mushrooms, salt, and thyme. Cook, stirring occasionally, until the mushrooms are deeply browned, about 5 minutes.

3. Add the cream cheese and cook, stirring, until it melts, a few minutes more.

4. Spoon the mushroom mixture on the eggplant slices and roll the eggplant around the filling. Place the eggplant rolls seam-side down in the baking dish.

5. Bake, uncovered, until the eggplant is soft and golden, about 45 minutes.

INGREDIENT TIP: Remove the bitter fluids from eggplant by placing the slices in a colander and salting them. Allow them to sit and drain for 20 minutes before rinsing away excess salt and patting them dry.

PER SERVING: Calories: 139; Total fat: 8g; Sodium: 487mg; Carbohydrates: 12g; Fiber: 4g; Protein: 7g

These pitas are easy to customize with your own favorite GERD-friendly ingredients. They make a delicious and quick vegetarian meal on the go, so they're perfect for lunch or a quick weekday dinner or breakfast. The fennel is especially beneficial for acid reflux, and it adds a lovely crunch to the sandwich.

VEGGIE PITAS

SERVES: 4 • **PREP TIME:** 10 minutes

VEGETARIAN

4 pitas, halved
8 tablespoons fat-free cream cheese
1 (14-ounce) can artichoke hearts, drained and chopped
½ fennel bulb, very thinly sliced
2 cups baby spinach

1. Spread 1 tablespoon of cream cheese in each of the pita halves.

2. Stuff each with the artichokes, fennel slices, and baby spinach.

SUBSTITUTION TIP: Make this vegan by replacing the cream cheese with Guacamole (page 30).

PER SERVING: Calories: 216; Total fat: 2g; Sodium: 566mg; Carbohydrates: 38g; Fiber: 9g; Protein: 13g

This take on mac and cheese is lower in fat, so it won't aggravate your GERD, but it still allows you to enjoy the cheesy goodness. It's also easy to make this vegan and gluten-free depending on your own dietary needs and restrictions (see the Substitution Tip).

PASTA WITH CAULIFLOWER SAUCE

SERVES: 4 · **PREP TIME:** 10 minutes · **COOK TIME:** 5 minutes

VEGETARIAN

2 cups cauliflower florets, boiled and drained
¼ cup nonfat milk
½ teaspoon sea salt
½ cup nonfat grated Cheddar cheese
8 ounces whole-wheat elbow macaroni, cooked according to package instructions and drained

1. In a large pot, combine the cooked and drained cauliflower, milk, and salt. Bring just to a boil.

2. Pour the cauliflower mixture into a blender or food processor and add the cheese. Blend until smooth.

3. Pour over the hot, cooked pasta.

SUBSTITUTION TIP: You can make this vegan by replacing the milk with nondairy milk and the Cheddar cheese with any low-fat vegan cheese. Use gluten-free pasta to make it gluten-free as well.

PER SERVING: Calories: 230; Total fat: 0g; Sodium: 480mg; Carbohydrates: 45g; Fiber: 6g; Protein: 11g

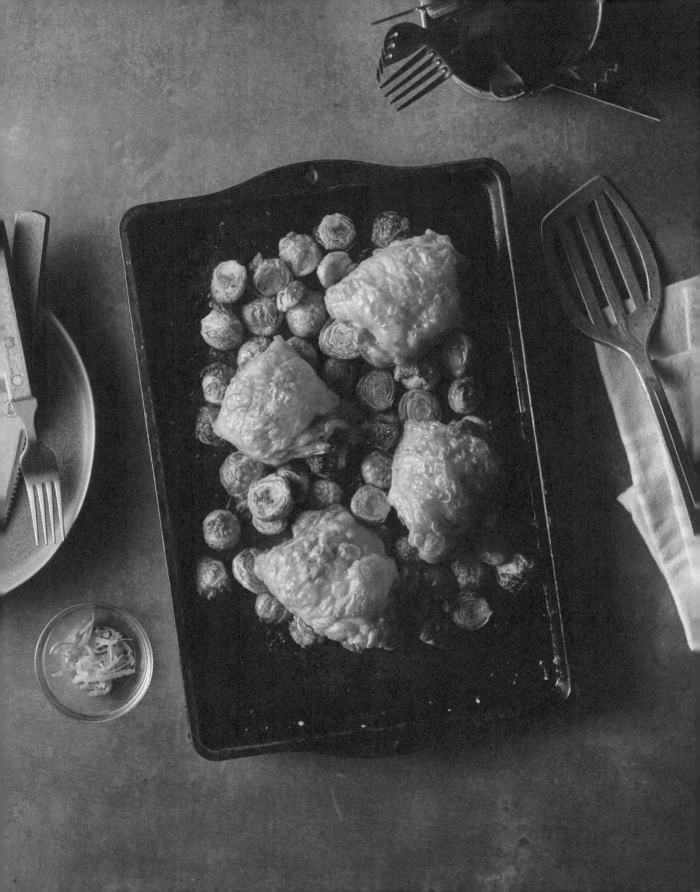

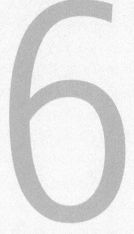

Seafood and Poultry

Scallops have a sweet, mild flavor, and they cook very quickly. The baby spinach makes a great side dish, and because you cook it in the same pan as the scallops, cleanup is minimal. The orange zest adds citrus flavor without the acid.

PAN-SEARED SCALLOPS WITH SPINACH

SERVES: 4 • **PREP TIME:** 5 minutes • **COOK TIME:** 10 minutes

GLUTEN-FREE
LOW-FODMAP

2 tablespoons olive oil
12 ounces sea scallops
½ teaspoon sea salt, divided
3 cups baby spinach
Zest of ½ orange

1. Place a large nonstick skillet over medium-high heat and add the olive oil.

2. Season the scallops with ¼ teaspoon of salt.

3. Once the oil shimmers, place the scallops in the pan. Cook until browned on each side, 2 to 3 minutes per side.

4. Using tongs, transfer the scallops to a platter. Tent with aluminum foil to keep warm.

5. Add the spinach, orange zest, and remaining ¼ teaspoon of salt to the pan.

6. Cook, stirring often, until the spinach wilts, about 3 minutes.

INGREDIENT TIP: Prepare the scallops before cooking by removing the small tendon that runs along the side of the scallop with a sharp paring knife.

PER SERVING: *Calories: 144; Total fat: 8g; Sodium: 454mg; Carbohydrates: 4g; Fiber: 1g; Protein: 15g*

Instead of breading and frying the shrimp as you would in a traditional coconut shrimp dish, this recipe is a stir-fry with a little coconut added. It gives you the sweet flavors without all the fat that activates GERD. The ginger and honey are also both soothing for GERD. Serve this with a side of steamed brown rice and some steamed veggies for a delicious full meal.

COCONUT-GINGER SHRIMP

SERVES: 4 · **PREP TIME:** 5 minutes · **COOK TIME:** 10 minutes

GLUTEN-FREE

2 tablespoons coconut oil

12 ounces medium shrimp, peeled, deveined, and tails off

2 tablespoons unsweetened coconut flakes

1 teaspoon grated fresh ginger

1 tablespoon honey

½ teaspoon sea salt

1. Place a large nonstick skillet over medium-high heat and add the coconut oil. Once the oil shimmers, add the shrimp, coconut flakes, and ginger. Cook, stirring often, until the shrimp turns pink, about 7 minutes.

2. Add the honey and salt. Cook, stirring, for 1 minute more.

SUBSTITUTION TIP: To make this low-FODMAP, omit the honey. Instead, add a few drops of liquid stevia.

PER SERVING: Calories: 200; Total fat: 10g; Sodium: 760mg; Carbohydrates: 5g; Fiber: <1g; Protein: 21g

You can use either aluminum foil or parchment paper to make these packets of fish and veggies. Either works well to seal in the moisture as you cook the fish, so the veggies and fish come out perfectly steamed. The thinner you slice the fennel, the more tender it is, so if you prefer your fennel with a little crisp remaining, cut thicker slices.

COD AND FENNEL PACKETS

SERVES: 4 • **PREP TIME:** 5 minutes • **COOK TIME:** 20 minutes

GLUTEN-FREE
LOW-FODMAP

4 (4-ounce) cod fillets
1 tablespoon olive oil
1 fennel bulb, thinly sliced
2 tablespoons chopped fennel fronds
½ teaspoon sea salt
1 teaspoon grated lemon zest
½ cup vegetable broth, store-bought or Home-made Vegetable Broth (page 114)

1. Preheat the oven to 400°F.

2. Lay out four large pieces of aluminum foil or parchment paper. Place a cod fillet in the center of each. Brush the fish with olive oil, or drizzle oil over the fillets. Top each fillet with the fennel slices and fronds and sprinkle with the salt and lemon zest. Drizzle with more olive oil.

3. Fold into packets, leaving an opening at the top. Place on a rimmed baking sheet.

4. Pour 2 tablespoons of vegetable broth in each packet; then seal it closed.

5. Bake until the fish is flaky and opaque, about 20 minutes.

FLAVOR BOOST: Add up to ¼ of a sliced red bell pepper with the fennel to add color and flavor.

PER SERVING: Calories: 169; Total fat: 5g; Sodium: 412mg; Carbohydrates: 5g; Fiber: 2g; Protein: 26g

Dill and fish go perfectly together, and this recipe is so quick and easy. It uses a little bit of lemon zest to give you citrus flavors without the acid. Make it a meal by serving it with Shredded Brussels Sprouts (page 36) or a simple side of steamed veggies.

LEMON-DILL BAKED COD

SERVES: 4 · **PREP TIME:** 5 minutes · **COOK TIME:** 12 minutes

GLUTEN-FREE
LOW-FODMAP

4 (4-ounce) cod fillets
2 tablespoons chopped
   fresh dill
1 teaspoon grated
   lemon zest
½ teaspoon sea salt
1 tablespoon olive oil

1. Preheat the oven to 400°F. Line a rimmed baking sheet with parchment paper.

2. Place the cod on the prepared baking sheet and sprinkle with the dill, lemon zest, and salt. Drizzle with the olive oil.

3. Bake until the fish is flaky and opaque, 10 to 12 minutes.

FLAVOR BOOST: Increase the olive oil to 2 tablespoons and mix it with the dill, lemon zest, salt, and ½ cup of panko bread crumbs. Sprinkle over the fish before baking.

PER SERVING: *Calories: 149; Total fat: 4g; Sodium: 379mg; Carbohydrates: <1g; Fiber: <1g; Protein: 25g*

Serve these simple crab cakes with a side of Guacamole (page 30), or layer the crab cakes and avocado spread in a pita. Baking eliminates some of the fat typically found in fried crab cakes, and alkaline cilantro adds fresh flavors to the finished crab cakes.

CRAB CAKES

SERVES: 4 · **PREP TIME:** 5 minutes, plus 30 minutes to chill · **COOK TIME:** 15 minutes

12 ounces lump crab meat, drained
1 cup panko bread crumbs
¼ cup chopped fresh cilantro
1 large egg, beaten
Zest of 1 lime
½ teaspoon sea salt
Nonstick cooking spray

1. In a medium bowl, combine the crab, panko bread crumbs, cilantro, egg, lime zest, and salt and mix well. Cover and refrigerate for 30 minutes.

2. Preheat the oven to 450°F. Spray a rimmed baking sheet with nonstick cooking spray.

3. Form the mixture into four crab cakes and place on the baking sheet. Bake until golden, about 15 minutes.

INGREDIENT TIP: When working with lump crab meat, always drain it in a colander, pat it dry, and then pick it over to make sure it doesn't have any bits of shell in it.

PER SERVING: *Calories: 203; Total fat: 2g; Sodium: 672mg; Carbohydrates: 19g; Fiber: 1g; Protein: 24g*

The great part about this fish stew is you can jazz it up with more veggies (carrots or butternut squash are delicious here), and you can use just one type of fish or add different types of fish and shellfish to make it even more interesting. For example, use 6 ounces each of cod and shrimp.

SIMPLE FISH STEW

SERVES: 4 · **PREP TIME:** 5 minutes · **COOK TIME:** 10 minutes

2 tablespoons olive oil

1 fennel bulb, chopped

12 ounces cod, halibut, or white fish, skin removed and cut into bite-size pieces

2 tablespoons all-purpose flour

3 cups vegetable broth, store-bought or Homemade Vegetable Broth (page 114)

½ teaspoon sea salt

2 tablespoons chopped fennel fronds

1. Place a large pot over medium-high heat and add the olive oil. Once the oil shimmers, add the fennel bulb and cook, stirring occasionally, until the fennel starts to soften, about 5 minutes.

2. Add the fish and cook until opaque, about 3 minutes more.

3. Add the flour and cook, stirring carefully to not break up the pieces of fish, for 1 minute.

4. Add the broth and the salt. Cook, stirring often, until it thickens, 2 to 3 minutes.

5. Stir in the fennel fronds just before serving.

FLAVOR BOOST: Add ½ red bell pepper, chopped, when you add the fennel bulb and then add ½ cup of corn kernels when you add the broth and salt.

PER SERVING: Calories: 187; Total fat: 8g; Sodium: 395mg; Carbohydrates: 9g; Fiber: 2g; Protein: 21g

The honey, ginger, orange, and soy glaze blends beautifully with the pink flesh of the salmon in this simple dish. Honey and ginger are both especially soothing for acid reflux. It's easy to make this gluten-free by using gluten-free tamari or coconut aminos in place of the low-sodium soy sauce.

HONEY-SOY SALMON

SERVES: 4 • **PREP TIME:** 5 minutes • **COOK TIME:** 12 minutes

Nonstick cooking spray
2 tablespoons low-sodium soy sauce
2 tablespoons honey
Zest of ½ orange
1 tablespoon grated fresh ginger
4 (4-ounce) salmon fillets

1. Preheat the oven to 450°F. Spray a rimmed baking sheet with nonstick cooking spray.

2. In a small bowl, whisk together the soy sauce, honey, orange zest, and ginger.

3. Place the salmon fillets on the prepared baking sheet and brush with the honey-soy mixture.

4. Bake until the fish is flaky and opaque, about 12 minutes.

INGREDIENT TIP: Cook the fillets with the skin on (skin-side down), and then remove the skin before serving. The skin imparts flavor, but removing it allows you to minimize the fat in this dish, which is helpful for minimizing acid reflux.

PER SERVING: Calories: 201; Total fat: 7g; Sodium: 338mg; Carbohydrates: 10g; Fiber: <1g; Protein: 23g

Adding fish sauce to both the ground turkey and the spread brings big umami flavors to these delicious turkey burgers. Serve them in a bun or a pita or, if you like, in a lettuce wrap for a gluten-free sandwich.

TURKEY BURGERS

SERVES: 4 • **PREP TIME:** 10 minutes • **COOK TIME:** 10 minutes

12 ounces 93 percent lean ground turkey

1 teaspoon fish sauce, divided

½ teaspoon sea salt

2 tablespoons grated fresh ginger, divided

Olive oil spray

½ cup plain nonfat yogurt

4 whole-wheat hamburger buns, toasted

1. In a large bowl, combine the ground turkey with ½ teaspoon of fish sauce, the salt, and 1 tablespoon of ginger and mix well. Form the mixture into four patties.

2. Spray a large nonstick skillet with olive oil spray and place over medium-high heat. Once the pan is hot, add the turkey patties and cook until browned, about 5 minutes per side.

3. While the patties cook, in a small bowl whisk together the yogurt with the remaining ½ teaspoon of fish sauce and 1 tablespoon of ginger. Spread this on the toasted buns.

4. Add the cooked turkey burgers and serve.

FLAVOR BOOST: Add the zest of 1 lime, ¼ cup of chopped fresh cilantro, and ½ teaspoon of low-sodium soy sauce to the yogurt to add even more flavor to these burgers.

PER SERVING: Calories: 266; Total fat: 8g; Sodium: 680mg; Carbohydrates: 27g; Fiber: 4g; Protein: 24g

Serve this stir-fry with Fried Rice (page 66) or with Peanut Butter Noodles (page 54) and some steamed veggies for a full, GERD-friendly meal. The ginger and carrots are both especially soothing to acid reflux, and it's easy to make this dish gluten-free by using coconut aminos or tamari in place of the soy sauce.

GROUND TURKEY STIR-FRY

SERVES: 4 • **PREP TIME:** 5 minutes • **COOK TIME:** 10 minutes

2 tablespoons olive oil

12 ounces 93 percent lean ground turkey

4 carrots, peeled and grated

1 tablespoon grated fresh ginger

1 tablespoon low-sodium soy sauce

1. Place a large nonstick skillet over medium-high heat and add the olive oil. Once the oil shimmers, add the turkey and cook, using a wooden spoon to break the meat into smaller pieces, until browned, about 5 minutes.

2. Add the carrots and ginger. Cook, stirring often, until the carrots soften, about 3 minutes more.

3. Add the soy sauce and cook for 1 minute more.

FLAVOR BOOST: Add 1 cup of fresh or frozen peas to the stir-fry when you add the carrots.

PER SERVING: *Calories: 209; Total fat: 13g; Sodium: 250mg; Carbohydrates: 6g; Fiber: 2g; Protein: 17g*

Cooking the turkey breast with the skin on keeps the meat moist, but you'll want to remove the skin before serving since poultry skin is high in fat, which can aggravate GERD. While this takes a while to cook, it's passive time; most of the time the turkey breast is in the oven roasting, leaving you free to make simple side dishes or mingle with family and guests.

SAGE-BAKED TURKEY BREAST

SERVES: 6 · **PREP TIME:** 5 minutes · **COOK TIME:** 90 minutes

GLUTEN-FREE
LOW-FODMAP

1 teaspoon sea salt
1 teaspoon ground sage
1 tablespoon olive oil
Zest of 1 lemon
1 whole skin-on
  turkey breast

1. Preheat the oven to 350°F. Place a roasting rack in a roasting pan.

2. In a small bowl, whisk together the salt, sage, oil, and lemon zest.

3. Pull the skin away from the turkey breast (leaving it attached) and rub the sage mixture on the meat under the skin. Put the breast in the roasting pan.

4. Bake until the breast reads 165°F on an instant-read thermometer, about 90 minutes.

5. Transfer the turkey breast to a cutting board and tent it with aluminum foil. Let rest for 20 minutes before carving.

INGREDIENT TIP: Rinse the turkey breast and pat it dry with paper towels before seasoning and cooking it.

PER SERVING: Calories: 165; Total fat: 3g; Sodium: 451mg; Carbohydrates: <1g; Fiber: <1g; Protein: 32g

These chicken fingers are tasty by themselves, delicious on salads, and yummy in sandwiches. You can make them gluten-free and low-FODMAP by using gluten-free bread crumbs and gluten-free flour. Try serving them with Guacamole (page 30) or Ginger-Cilantro Yogurt Spread/Dip (page 123) as a dipping sauce.

BAKED CHICKEN FINGERS

SERVES: 4 • **PREP TIME:** 5 minutes • **COOK TIME:** 20 minutes

2 large eggs
1 cup panko bread crumbs
¼ cup all-purpose flour
1 tablespoon dried Italian herbs
½ teaspoon sea salt
12 ounces chicken tenders or boneless, skinless chicken breast, cut into ½-inch-thick strips

1. Preheat the oven to 425°F.

2. In one bowl, beat the eggs. In another bowl, whisk together the panko bread crumbs, flour, herbs, and salt.

3. Dip the chicken strips in the beaten eggs and then in the bread crumb mixture, gently shaking off any excess. Place on a rimmed baking sheet.

4. Bake until the chicken is cooked through and the coating is golden brown, about 20 minutes.

BATCH IT: These will freeze well and reheat in the microwave, so feel free to make a double or triple batch. Freeze extras in 3-ounce servings in zip-top bags for up to 6 months.

PER SERVING: *Calories: 230; Total fat: 4g; Sodium: 503mg; Carbohydrates: 25g; Fiber: 2g; Protein: 24g*

Poaching chicken breast keeps it moist while imparting the flavors of the herbs in the poaching liquid to the chicken. You can eat the chicken hot when it comes out of the liquid, or you can shred it and save it for sandwiches, salads, and more. It will keep in the freezer for up to 6 months.

HERB-POACHED CHICKEN

SERVES: 4 · **PREP TIME:** 5 minutes · **COOK TIME:** 12 minutes

GLUTEN-FREE
LOW-FODMAP

4 cups chicken broth, store-bought or Home-made Chicken Broth (page 116)
1 sprig fresh rosemary
1 sprig fresh thyme
½ teaspoon sea salt
4 (4-ounce) boneless, skinless chicken breasts

1. In a large pot, combine all the ingredients.

2. Place the pot over medium-high heat and bring to a boil. Reduce the temperature to low and cover. Cook until the chicken reads 165°F on an instant-read thermometer, about 12 minutes.

3. Slice before serving.

INGREDIENT TIP: There's no need to strip the herbs off their sprigs. Instead, just rinse them and put them in the pot whole. For a more intense flavor, add two sprigs of each herb along with a bay leaf.

PER SERVING: *Calories: 144; Total fat: 4g; Sodium: 491mg; Carbohydrates: 3g; Fiber: <1g; Protein: 26g*

Cook the thighs with the skin on, and then, before serving, remove the skin to minimize fat. The fat from the skin will trickle onto the Brussels sprouts, making them tender and delicious. Feel free to add additional GERD-friendly herbs to the lemon zest and salt that you sprinkle on the chicken, such as Italian herbs or ground sage.

BAKED CHICKEN THIGHS WITH BRUSSELS SPROUTS

SERVES: 4 • **PREP TIME:** 10 minutes • **COOK TIME:** 1 hour

GLUTEN-FREE
LOW-FODMAP

12 ounces Brussels sprouts, halved
4 whole bone-in, skin-on chicken thighs
½ teaspoon sea salt
1 teaspoon grated lemon zest

1. Preheat the oven to 425°F.

2. Place the Brussels sprouts, cut-side down, in a single layer on the bottom of a 9-by-13-inch baking dish.

3. Rub the sea salt and lemon zest under the skin of the chicken thighs. Put the thighs on top of the Brussels sprouts.

4. Bake until the chicken reads 165°F on an instant-read thermometer, about 1 hour.

5. Remove the skin before serving.

FLAVOR BOOST: Sprinkle the cooked Brussels sprouts with up to ¼ cup of grated Parmesan cheese, but don't add much more than this because it can activate GERD.

PER SERVING: *Calories: 145; Total fat: 6g; Sodium: 525mg; Carbohydrates: 8g; Fiber: 3g; Protein: 16g*

Cashews add crunch to this coconut and ginger chicken. Serve on top of steamed rice with a side of veggies, or add veggies to the chicken stir-fry to make it a more complete meal (see the Flavor Boost). This will keep well, so you can make a larger batch and freeze it for meals on the go or for use after a particularly busy day.

CASHEW CHICKEN

SERVES: 4 · **PREP TIME:** 10 minutes · **COOK TIME:** 10 minutes

GLUTEN-FREE

2 tablespoons olive oil

12 ounces boneless, skinless chicken breast, cut into 1-inch pieces

1 tablespoon grated fresh ginger

1 cup light coconut milk

½ teaspoon sea salt

½ cup chopped cashews

1. Place a large nonstick skillet over medium-high heat and add the olive oil. Once the oil shimmers, add the chicken and ginger and cook, stirring occasionally, until the chicken is opaque, about 7 minutes.

2. Add the coconut milk and salt. Bring to a simmer. Cook until heated through, about 2 minutes.

3. Sprinkle with the chopped cashews before serving.

FLAVOR BOOST: Add 2 sliced carrots, 1 cup of broccoli florets, and ½ sliced red bell pepper. To incorporate, remove the browned chicken from the pan with a slotted spoon and add the vegetables. Cook, stirring often, until they are crisp-tender, about 5 minutes. Return the chicken to the pan and add the coconut milk, salt, and cashews.

PER SERVING: Calories: 280; Total fat: 21g; Sodium: 455mg; Carbohydrates: 7g; Fiber: 1g; Protein: 21g

This is essentially a quick chicken stir-fry. The trick to flavorful mushrooms on the stove top is to cook them without stirring for about 5 minutes so they begin to brown, which brings out deep flavors. You can also replace the rice with cauliflower rice if you prefer, which adds nice alkalinity that is beneficial for acid reflux. To make this lower in FODMAPs, use oyster mushrooms instead of cremini mushrooms.

EASY CHICKEN AND RICE WITH MUSHROOMS

SERVES: 4 · **PREP TIME:** 10 minutes · **COOK TIME:** 15 minutes

GLUTEN-FREE

2 tablespoons olive oil
12 ounces boneless, skinless chicken breast, cut into 1-inch pieces
8 ounces cremini mushrooms, halved
1 teaspoon dried thyme
½ teaspoon sea salt
1 cup cooked brown rice

1. Place a large nonstick skillet over medium-high heat and add the olive oil. Once the oil shimmers, add the chicken and cook, stirring occasionally, until it is opaque, about 7 minutes. Using a slotted spoon, transfer the chicken to a plate and set aside.

2. Add the mushrooms to the pan and sprinkle them with the thyme and salt. Cook, stirring occasionally, until the mushrooms are well browned, about 5 minutes.

3. Return the chicken to the pan along with any juices that have collected on the plate. Add the cooked rice. Cook, stirring often, until everything is heated through, 2 to 3 minutes.

INGREDIENT TIP: To clean the mushrooms, don't submerge or rinse them, which will waterlog them. Instead, use a soft brush or paper towel to wipe away any traces of dirt.

PER SERVING: Calories: 211; Total fat: 10g; Sodium: 429mg; Carbohydrates: 13g; Fiber: 2g; Protein: 20g

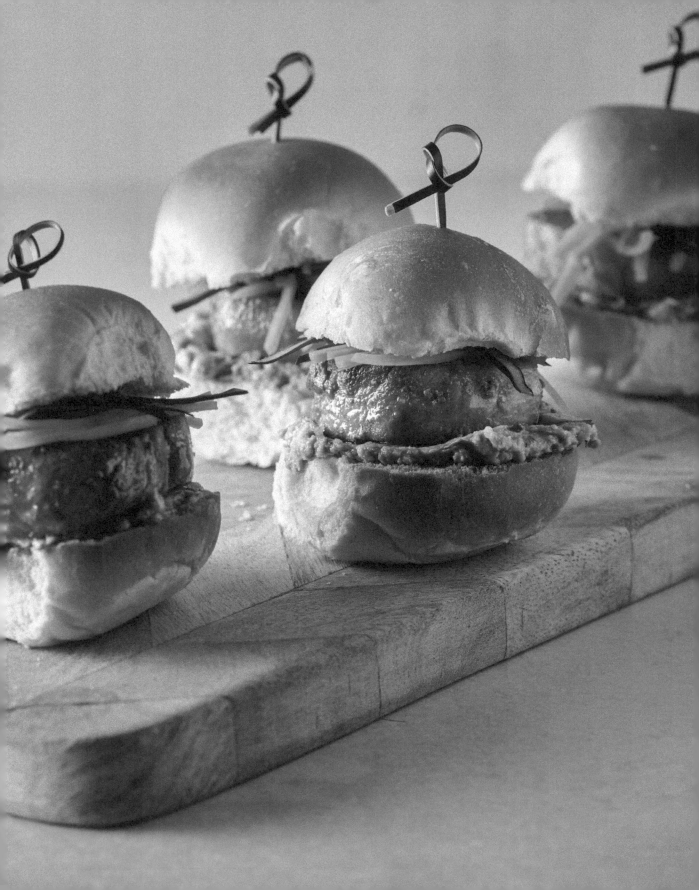

7

Pork, Beef, and Lamb

Be sure you use red apples in this quick skillet meal, because they are far more GERD-friendly than their tart green counterparts. Save time by purchasing pre-shredded cabbage (coleslaw mix) in the produce section of your grocery store. Filled with flavorful acid reflux–friendly ingredients, this makes a delicious, savory, and quick dinner.

PORK AND RED APPLE SKILLET

SERVES: 6 · **PREP TIME:** 10 minutes · **COOK TIME:** 15 minutes

GLUTEN-FREE

2 tablespoons olive oil
1 pound pork tenderloin, cut into 1-inch pieces
2 red apples, peeled and chopped
1 head cabbage, shredded
1 tablespoon grated fresh ginger
½ teaspoon sea salt

1. Place a large nonstick skillet over medium-high heat and add the olive oil. Once the oil shimmers, add the pork and cook, stirring occasionally, until browned, about 5 minutes.

2. Using a slotted spoon, remove the pork from the fat in the pan and place on a plate. Tent with a piece of aluminum foil to keep warm.

3. Add the apples to the fat in the pan and cook, stirring occasionally, until crisp-tender, about 4 minutes.

4. Add the cabbage, ginger, and salt. Cook, stirring often, for 2 minutes. Return the pork to the pan. Cook for 2 minutes more.

SUBSTITUTION TIP: Make this lower in FODMAPs by replacing the red apple with 1 bulb of jicama, peeled and chopped.

PER SERVING: Calories: 189; Total fat: 9g; Sodium: 245mg; Carbohydrates: 15g; Fiber: 5g; Protein: 15g

Pork tenderloin is lean and flavorful. The maple glaze adds a ton of flavor and beneficial ginger to help soothe GERD. Serve it with steamed rice, a baked potato, or a simple side salad for a delicious and satisfying meal. Leftovers of the pork make a great salad topper—it will keep in an airtight container in the refrigerator for up to 4 days.

MAPLE-GLAZED PORK LOIN

SERVES: 6 · **PREP TIME:** 10 minutes · **COOK TIME:** 20 minutes

GLUTEN-FREE
LOW-FODMAP

1 tablespoon olive oil
¼ cup pure maple syrup
1 tablespoon grated fresh ginger
1 teaspoon cinnamon
½ teaspoon sea salt
1 (1½-pound) pork tenderloin

1. Preheat the oven to 450°F. Place a roasting rack in a roasting pan.

2. In a small bowl, whisk together the olive oil, syrup, ginger, cinnamon, and salt. Brush this mixture all over the tenderloin. Place the pork on the roasting rack.

3. Bake until the pork reads 145°F on an instant-read thermometer, 15 to 20 minutes.

4. Transfer the pork to a cutting board. Tent a piece of aluminum foil for at least 10 minutes before carving.

INGREDIENT TIP: If you have leftover glaze after brushing it on the pork, bring the remaining glaze to a boil in a small pot over medium-high heat and simmer for 5 minutes. Serve spooned over the cooked pork.

PER SERVING: *Calories: 186; Total fat: 7g; Sodium: 231mg; Carbohydrates: 10g; Fiber: <1g; Protein: 19g*

Rosemary and pork go beautifully together, and the orange zest and honey complement the herb, giving this recipe a sweet and savory balance. Honey is also soothing for GERD, unless you also have FODMAP issues; if you do, see the Substitution Tip for a lower-FODMAP alternative. The trick with pork chops is to avoid overcooking them, so check them after about 15 minutes with an instant-read thermometer. If the temperature is 140°F or higher, remove them from the oven, tent them with aluminum foil, and let them rest for 10 minutes to bring the temperature up to 145°F.

ROSEMARY-BAKED PORK CHOPS

SERVES: 4 · **PREP TIME:** 10 minutes · **COOK TIME:** 20 minutes

GLUTEN-FREE

2 tablespoons olive oil

2 tablespoons honey

2 tablespoons chopped fresh rosemary or 2 teaspoons dried rosemary

1 teaspoon grated orange zest

½ teaspoon sea salt

4 (1-inch-thick) bone-in pork chops

1. Preheat the oven to 375°F. Line a rimmed baking sheet with parchment paper.

2. In a small bowl, whisk together the olive oil, honey, rosemary, orange zest, and salt. Brush the oil mixture on both sides of the pork chops and place them on the baking sheet.

3. Bake until the chops read 145°F on an instant-read thermometer, 15 to 20 minutes.

4. Tent the pork chops with a piece of aluminum foil and let rest for 10 minutes before serving.

SUBSTITUTION TIP: Make this lower in FODMAPs by replacing the honey with 2 tablespoons of brown sugar and 1 tablespoon of broth or water.

PER SERVING: Calories: 232; Total fat: 14g; Sodium: 697mg; Carbohydrates: 10g; Fiber: <1g; Protein: 17g

Pork chops have a tendency to dry out, but adding gravy is a great way to keep them moist and delicious. If you are sensitive to gluten and/or FODMAPs, you can adjust this by using gluten-free flour in place of the all-purpose flour.

PAN-SEARED PORK CHOPS WITH GRAVY

SERVES: 4 • **PREP TIME:** 10 minutes • **COOK TIME:** 15 minutes

2 tablespoons olive oil

4 (1-inch-thick) bone-in pork chops

1 teaspoon sea salt, divided

1 teaspoon dried thyme

3 tablespoons all-purpose flour

3 cups chicken or vegetable broth, store-bought or homemade (see page 116 or 114)

1. Place a large skillet over medium-high heat and add the olive oil.

2. Season the pork chops on both sides with ½ teaspoon of salt and the thyme.

3. Once the oil shimmers, add the chops to the pan and sear until an instant-read thermometer reads 145°F, about 5 minutes per side.

4. Using tongs, remove the pork from the fat and transfer to a platter. Tent the chops with a piece of aluminum foil.

5. With the pan still on the heat, add the flour to the fat in the pan and cook, stirring constantly, for 1 minute.

6. Pour in the broth and use the side of a spoon to scrape any browned bits from the bottom of the pan. Add the remaining ½ teaspoon of salt. Cook, stirring often, until the gravy thickens, 2 to 3 minutes.

7. Serve the chops with the gravy.

FLAVOR BOOST: Make a mushroom gravy by soaking 2 ounces of dried porcini mushrooms in the 3 cups of chicken broth, making sure the broth is very hot before soaking the mushrooms. Soak for 30 minutes and then strain out the mushrooms, reserving both the mushrooms and the broth. Chop the mushrooms and return them to the pan along with the hot broth to make your gravy.

PER SERVING: Calories: 242; Total fat: 15g; Sodium: 1,002mg; Carbohydrates: 7g; Fiber: <1g; Protein: 19g

These basic sliders make a tasty meal. You can add texture by topping them with shredded cabbage or grated carrots, which will add flavor and crunch. Use soft corn tortillas and top them with shredded lettuce and cooked corn to make a yummy taco variation of the basic recipe.

PORK SLIDERS

SERVES: 4 · **PREP TIME:** 10 minutes · **COOK TIME:** 10 minutes

2 tablespoons olive oil
1 pound pork ten-
  derloin, sliced into
  1-inch-thick pieces
1 teaspoon sea salt, divided
½ avocado
2 tablespoons chopped
  fresh cilantro
8 slider buns, toasted

1. Place a large nonstick skillet over medium-high heat and add the olive oil.

2. Season the pork slices all over with ½ teaspoon of salt.

3. Once the oil shimmers, add the pork to the pan and cook until an instant-read thermometer reads 145°F, about 4 minutes per side.

4. In a small bowl, mash together the avocado, the remaining ½ teaspoon of salt, and the cilantro.

5. Spread the avocado mash on the buns. Top with the pork slices.

FLAVOR BOOST: Replace the mashed avocado with ½ cup of nonfat plain yogurt. Omit the cilantro and instead grate 1 red apple (peeled and cored) to mix in with the yogurt and serve as a topping for the sliders.

PER SERVING: *Calories: 417; Total fat: 17g; Sodium: 914mg; Carbohydrates: 39g; Fiber: 4g; Protein: 33g*

A 12-cup muffin tin is the perfect vessel for cooking these mini meatloaves, yielding a perfect serving from two muffins. Fish sauce adds a ton of flavor to the meat, giving the muffins a delicious burst of umami while the grated carrots have enough alkalinity to be soothing to acid reflux.

MINI MEATLOAVES

SERVES: 6 · **PREP TIME:** 10 minutes · **COOK TIME:** 30 minutes

*12 ounces extra-lean
   ground beef*
½ cup skim milk
½ cup bread crumbs
1 carrot, grated
1 tablespoon fish sauce
½ teaspoon sea salt

1. Preheat the oven to 350°F.

2. In a large bowl, mix together all the ingredients. Scoop the mixture into a 12-cup muffin tin.

3. Bake until the mini meatloaves read 165°F on an instant-read thermometer, about 30 minutes.

SUBSTITUTION TIP: Make this gluten-free and lower in FODMAPs by using gluten-free bread crumbs in place of regular bread crumbs.

PER SERVING (2 MUFFINS): Calories: 106; Total fat: 2g; Sodium: 480mg; Carbohydrates: 8g; Fiber: 1g; Protein: 14g

There's no need to give up taco night if you have GERD. With a few simple substitutions, you can still enjoy the flavor of tacos without the heartburn. Make the marinade and marinate the steak overnight or for up to 24 hours, and you have the perfect quick after-work recipe.

BEEF TACOS

SERVES: 4 • **PREP TIME:** 15 minutes, plus 4 hours to marinate • **COOK TIME:** 10 minutes

GLUTEN-FREE

2 tablespoons olive oil
½ cup chopped fresh cilantro
Zest of 1 lime
½ teaspoon sea salt
12 ounces skirt steak
4 soft corn tortillas, warmed

1. In a blender or food processor, combine the olive oil, cilantro, lime zest, and salt. Pour into a zip-top bag and add the skirt steak. Make sure the steak is coated with the marinade and refrigerate for at least 4 hours and up to 24 hours.

2. Preheat the oven's broiler to high. Place an oven rack in the highest position.

3. Remove the steak from the marinade and discard the marinade. Use a paper towel to wipe away excess marinade from the meat and place it on a broiling pan.

4. Broil for 3 to 4 minutes per side, until an instant-read thermometer reads 145°F.

5. Let the steak rest for 10 minutes on a cutting board. Then slice against the grain and serve on the corn tortillas.

FLAVOR BOOST: Add 1 teaspoon of ground cumin to the marinade. To serve, top the tacos with up to ¼ cup of grated fat-free Cheddar cheese and 2 tablespoons of Guacamole (page 30).

PER SERVING: Calories: 305; Total fat: 18g; Sodium: 364mg; Carbohydrates: 12g; Fiber: 2g; Protein: 23g

Blackberry and steak may sound like a strange combination, but it has a beautiful balance of sweet and savory. Alkaline blackberries are also good for your acid reflux, and the flavor brings out the meatiness of the steak.

SKIRT STEAK WITH BLACKBERRY THYME SAUCE

SERVES: 4 · **PREP TIME:** 15 minutes · **COOK TIME:** 15 minutes

GLUTEN-FREE

2 cups fresh black-
  berries or frozen
  blackberries, thawed
1 tablespoon chopped
  fresh thyme
½ teaspoon sea salt
¼ cup chicken or vegetable
  broth, store-bought
  or homemade
  (page 116 or 114)
12 ounces skirt steak

1. Preheat the oven's broiler to high. Place an oven rack in the highest position.

2. In a blender or food processor, combine the blackberries, thyme, salt, and broth. Blend until smooth.

3. Pour the mixture into a medium pot and place over medium-high heat. Bring to a simmer and cook until the sauce has thickened slightly, about 5 minutes.

4. Brush the blackberry sauce on both sides of the skirt steak. Place the steak on a broiling pan.

5. Broil for 3 to 4 minutes per side, until an instant-read thermometer reads 145°F.

6. Transfer the steak to a cutting board and let rest for 10 minutes. Then slice against the grain and serve.

SUBSTITUTION TIP: You can make this lower in FODMAPs by replacing the blackberries with the same amount of blueberries.

PER SERVING: Calories: 227; Total fat: 11g; Sodium: 356mg; Carbohydrates: 10g; Fiber: 4g; Protein: 23g

Fennel is one of the most acid reflux–friendly vegetables you can eat, and it adds a ton of anise flavor that's delicious with beef and mushrooms. Serve this dish over steamed rice or alongside roasted potatoes and steamed vegetables for a hearty and comforting meal.

BEEF, MUSHROOM, AND FENNEL SKILLET

SERVES: 4 · **PREP TIME:** 10 minutes · **COOK TIME:** 15 minutes

GLUTEN-FREE

2 tablespoons olive oil
12 ounces skirt steak, cut into 1-inch pieces
1 fennel bulb, chopped
8 ounces cremini mushrooms, quartered
1 teaspoon dried thyme
½ teaspoon sea salt
2 tablespoons chopped fennel fronds

1. Place a large nonstick skillet over medium-high heat and add the olive oil. Once the oil shimmers, add the beef and cook, stirring occasionally, until it is browned, 5 to 7 minutes.

2. Using tongs or a slotted spoon, remove the beef from the fat in the pan and transfer to a platter. Tent the platter with aluminum foil to keep warm.

3. Add the fennel bulb, mushrooms, thyme, and salt to the pan and cook, stirring occasionally, until the vegetables begin to brown, about 5 minutes.

4. Return the beef to the pan along with any juices that have collected on the platter. Cook, stirring often, until the beef is heated through, about 2 minutes. Remove the pan from the heat and stir in the fennel fronds.

———————————

SUBSTITUTION TIP: Make this lower in FODMAPs by replacing the cremini mushrooms with oyster mushrooms or omitting the mushrooms altogether and using 2 chopped carrots.

———————————

PER SERVING: Calories: 279; Total fat: 18g; Sodium: 389mg; Carbohydrates: 6g; Fiber: 3g; Protein: 25g

Broccoli and ginger are the perfect pairing with skirt steak, and they're great for acid reflux sufferers because of their soothing alkalinity. The flavors hold up well to the deep umami flavors of the beef. For more flavor, grate zest from ½ lime and add ¼ cup of chopped fresh cilantro to the stir-fry after you remove it from the heat.

SKIRT STEAK STIR-FRY

SERVES: 4 · **PREP TIME:** 10 minutes · **COOK TIME:** 15 minutes

GLUTEN-FREE
LOW FODMAP

2 tablespoons olive oil
12 ounces skirt steak, cut into ½-inch pieces
2 cups broccoli florets
1 tablespoon grated fresh ginger
1 tablespoon low-sodium soy sauce or tamari

1. Place a large nonstick skillet over medium-high heat and add the olive oil. Once the oil shimmers, add the steak and cook, stirring occasionally, until the beef is browned, 5 to 7 minutes.

2. Using a slotted spoon or tongs, remove the beef from the fat and transfer to a platter. Tent the platter with aluminum foil to keep warm.

3. Add the broccoli and ginger to the hot pan. Cook, stirring often, until the broccoli is tender, about 5 minutes.

4. Return the beef to the pan along with any juices that have collected on the platter. Add the soy sauce. Cook, stirring, until heated through, about 2 minutes more.

INGREDIENT TIP: Cut the skirt steak against the grain to shorten the fibers and make the meat much more tender.

PER SERVING: Calories: 266; Total fat: 17g; Sodium: 218mg; Carbohydrates: 3g; Fiber: 1g; Protein: 23g

This is a simple, flavorful, and basic stew that cooks very quickly. Jazz it up with more veggies, such as carrots, sweet potatoes, or potatoes, as well as herbs such as 1 teaspoon of dried thyme.

BEEF STEW

SERVES: 4 • **PREP TIME:** 10 minutes • **COOK TIME:** 15 minutes

2 tablespoons olive oil

12 ounces skirt steak, cut into ½-inch pieces

1 celery root, peeled and cut into ½-inch pieces

3 tablespoons all-purpose flour

4 cups chicken or vegetable broth, store-bought or homemade (page 116 or 114)

½ teaspoon sea salt

1. Place a large pot over medium-high heat and add the olive oil. Once the oil shimmers, add the beef and cook, stirring occasionally, until it is browned, 5 to 7 minutes.

2. Using tongs or a slotted spoon, remove the beef from the fat and transfer to a platter. Tent the platter with aluminum foil to keep warm.

3. Add the celery root to the pan and cook, stirring occasionally, until soft, about 4 minutes.

4. Add the flour and cook, stirring constantly, for 1 minute.

5. Add the broth and salt. Return the beef to the pot along with any juices that have collected on the platter. Bring to a simmer and cook, stirring occasionally, until the sauce thickens, about 3 minutes.

FLAVOR BOOST: Whisk 1 tablespoon of Dijon mustard into the broth before you add it to the pot. Don't add much more because it may aggravate acid reflux symptoms.

PER SERVING: *Calories: 321; Total fat: 18g; Sodium: 476mg; Carbohydrates: 17g; Fiber: 2g; Protein: 25g*

Whether you serve this over egg noodles or rice, this classic stroganoff recipe is hearty and warming. You can add 1 teaspoon of dried thyme for even more flavor or whisk in up to 1 tablespoon of Dijon mustard (but no more than that) to the broth and cornstarch mixture. Finish with chopped fresh parsley for a nice burst of color.

GROUND BEEF STROGANOFF

SERVES: 4 · **PREP TIME:** 10 minutes · **COOK TIME:** 15 minutes

GLUTEN-FREE

1 pound extra-lean ground beef
8 ounces cremini mushrooms, stems removed and caps quartered
½ teaspoon sea salt
3 cups chicken or vegetable broth, store-bought or homemade (see page 116 or 114)
2 tablespoons cornstarch
1 cup nonfat yogurt

1. Place a large nonstick skillet over medium-high heat and add the ground beef. Cook, breaking up the beef with a spoon, until it is browned, about 5 minutes.

2. Add the mushroom quarters and salt and cook, stirring occasionally, until the mushrooms are soft, about 4 minutes.

3. In a medium bowl, whisk together the broth and cornstarch. Add the mixture to the meat and mushrooms. Bring to a simmer and cook, stirring occasionally, until the sauce thickens, about 3 minutes.

4. Whisk in the yogurt and cook, stirring, until heated through, 1 to 2 minutes.

INGREDIENT TIP: Save the mushroom stems in a zip-top bag in the freezer. You can use them when you make Homemade Vegetable Broth.

PER SERVING: Calories: 211; Total fat: 5g; Sodium: 399mg; Carbohydrates: 12g; Fiber: 1g; Protein: 31g

The sweet and savory rub perfectly complements the flavor of the skirt steak. While broiling is a fast and easy option, you can also add smoky flavors by grilling the steak. To grill, heat the grill on high and oil the grate. Cook about 5 minutes per side.

DRY-RUBBED SKIRT STEAK

SERVES: 4 · **PREP TIME:** 5 minutes, plus 4 hours to marinate · **COOK TIME:** 10 minutes

GLUTEN-FREE
LOW-FODMAP

½ teaspoon sea salt
1 teaspoon ground cumin
1 teaspoon ground coriander
2 tablespoons brown sugar
1 tablespoon dried oregano
1 (12-ounce) skirt steak

1. In a small bowl, mix together the salt, cumin, coriander, brown sugar, and oregano.

2. Rub on both sides of the steak. Refrigerate for at least 4 hours and up to 24 hours.

3. Preheat the oven's broiler on high. Place an oven rack in the highest position.

4. Place the steak on a broiling pan.

5. Broil until an instant-read thermometer reads 145°F, about 4 minutes per side.

6. Transfer the steak to a cutting board. Let rest for 10 minutes; then slice against the grain and serve.

BATCH IT: Leftover dry-rubbed meat will keep well in the freezer in zip-top bags for up to 6 months. It can be reheated in the microwave to use on salads or in sandwiches.

PER SERVING: *Calories: 210; Total fat: 10g; Sodium: 358mg; Carbohydrates: 7g; Fiber: 1g; Protein: 23g*

Serve these meatballs with Tzatziki (page 128). The cooling cucumber yogurt is the perfect foil for these aromatically spiced lamb meatballs that are delicious on pitas, when served with rice, or even in some chicken broth to make a delicious soup.

MOROCCAN LAMB MEATBALLS

SERVES: 6 • **PREP TIME:** 5 minutes • **COOK TIME:** 45 minutes

GLUTEN-FREE
LOW-FODMAP

1 pound ground lamb
1 teaspoon ground cumin
1 teaspoon ground ginger
½ teaspoon ground allspice
½ teaspoon
  ground cinnamon
½ teaspoon sea salt

1. Preheat the oven to 400°F. Line a rimmed baking sheet with parchment paper.

2. In a large bowl, combine all the ingredients and mix well.

3. Form the mixture into 1-inch meatballs and place on the prepared baking sheet.

4. Bake until an instant-read thermometer reads 165°F, about 45 minutes.

_____

BATCH IT: These freeze beautifully and reheat in the microwave, so this is an excellent recipe to double or even triple so you can have quick meals on the go.

_____

PER SERVING: *Calories: 217; Total fat: 18g; Sodium: 239mg; Carbohydrates: 1g; Fiber: <1g; Protein: 13g*

Lamb loin chops (sometimes called lamb lollipops) are tender, delicious, and so quick and easy to cook. The herb paste that coats these chops pairs beautifully with the flavors of the lamb, and because the herbs are alkaline, they can also be quite GERD-friendly. Pair these chops with Maple-Ginger Roasted Beets (page 37) for a full meal.

HERBED LAMB CHOPS

SERVES: 6 • **PREP TIME:** 5 minutes • **COOK TIME:** 15 minutes

GLUTEN-FREE
LOW-FODMAP

*¼ cup chopped fresh
    Italian parsley*
*2 tablespoons chopped
    fresh rosemary*
*1 teaspoon grated
    lemon zest*
½ teaspoon sea salt
2 tablespoons olive oil
*1 pound bone-in lamb
    loin chops*

1. Preheat the oven to 400°F. Line a rimmed baking sheet with parchment paper.

2. In a blender or food processor, combine the parsley, rosemary, lemon zest, salt, and olive oil. Blend until well combined.

3. Place the lamb chops on the prepared baking sheet. Brush on both sides with the herb mixture.

4. Bake until an instant-read thermometer reads 145°F, 10 to 15 minutes.

FLAVOR BOOST: Add 1 tablespoon of Dijon mustard to the herb mixture to add flavor, but don't add much more than this since mustard in large amounts can aggravate GERD.

PER SERVING: *Calories: 110; Total fat: 8g; Sodium: 325mg; Carbohydrates: <1g; Fiber: <1g; Protein: 10g*

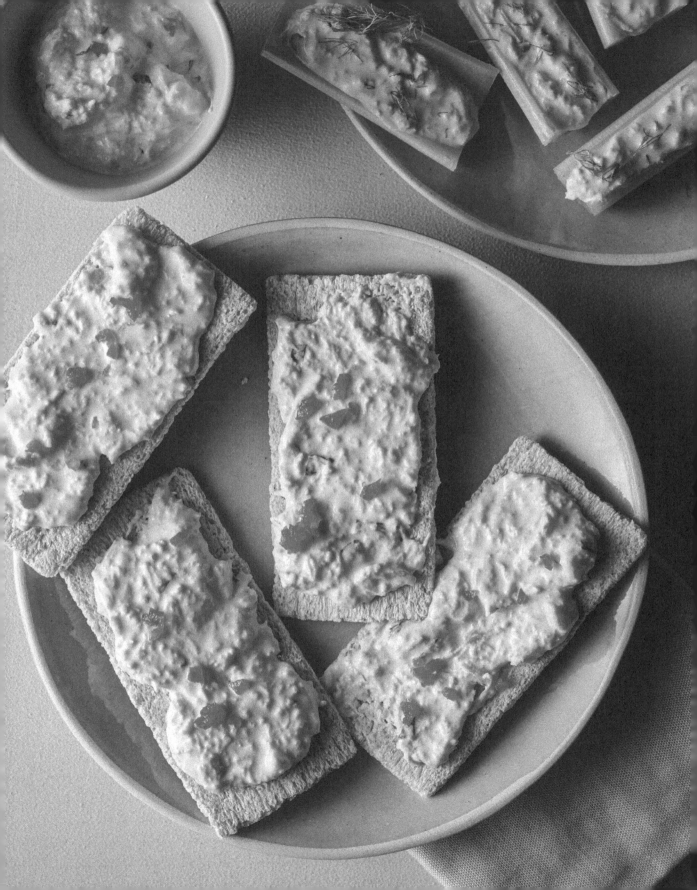

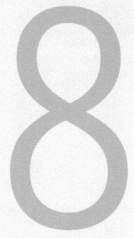

Broths, Sauces, and Condiments

The problem with traditional vegetable broth is that it's frequently made with onions, peppercorns, and garlic, which are all GERD triggers. This version has a mild flavor, but it's a great base for soups and sauces, and it won't trigger acid reflux. You can add additional herbs and spices for flavor depending on what you're using it for. For example, if you plan to make Vietnamese-style pho broth, add 2 (1-inch) pieces of fresh ginger and 2 star anise pods to the broth as it simmers. This broth doesn't have added salt, so you control the amount of salt that goes into your recipes.

HOMEMADE VEGETABLE BROTH

MAKES: 6 cups • **PREP TIME:** 5 minutes • **COOK TIME:** 2 hours

GLUTEN-FREE
VEGAN

8 cups water
3 carrots, roughly chopped
2 celery stalks,
   roughly chopped
8 ounces cremini mushrooms
2 sprigs fresh thyme

1. Combine all the ingredients in a large pot. Place over medium-high heat and bring to a boil. Reduce the heat to medium-low and simmer for 2 hours.

2. Alternatively, put all the ingredients in a 4- or 6-quart slow cooker. Cover and cook on low for 24 hours.

3. Strain through a sieve to remove the solids. Store in airtight containers in the refrigerator for up to 5 days or in the freezer for up to 6 months.

INGREDIENT TIP: Save vegetable trimmings such as fennel stalks, celery leaves, mushroom stems, and carrot peels to make stock. Store them in a zip-top bag in the freezer, put them in your pot, and cook them on low for 6 to 8 hours.

PER (1 CUP) SERVING: Calories: 8; Total fat: 0g; Sodium: 9mg; Carbohydrates: 2g; Fiber: 0g; Protein: <1g

Chicken bones and bony parts such as the neck, back, and wings make good chicken broth. Chicken feet also make really good chicken stock because they have lots of gelatin to give the broth lots of body. Use bones from a cooked chicken, such as a rotisserie chicken, to make broth. Don't skip defatting the broth in the final step, as this helps keep the fat in the broth from aggravating your acid reflux.

HOMEMADE CHICKEN BROTH

MAKES: 6 cups · **PREP TIME:** 5 minutes, plus chilling time · **COOK TIME:** 2 hours

GLUTEN-FREE

1 to 2 pounds chicken bones or chicken parts, such as wings and necks
3 carrots, roughly chopped
2 celery stalks, roughly chopped
2 sprigs fresh thyme
8 cups water

1. Combine all the ingredients in a large pot. Place over medium-high heat and bring to a boil. Reduce the heat to medium-low and simmer for 2 hours.

2. Alternatively, put all the ingredients in a 4- or 6-quart slow cooker. Cover and cook on low for 24 hours.

3. Strain through a sieve to remove the solids. Refrigerate for at least 8 hours.

4. Skim the fat off the top of the broth and discard it. Store in airtight containers in the refrigerator for up to 5 days or in the freezer for up to 6 months.

SUBSTITUTION TIP: Replace the chicken bones with turkey, pork, or beef bones to make various stocks. You can also make fish or shellfish stock using this recipe and replacing the chicken bones with shrimp or lobster shells or fish bones.

PER (1 CUP) SERVING: Calories: 33; Total fat: 1g; Sodium: 20mg; Carbohydrates: 3g; Fiber: 0g; Protein: 3g

This herb puree packs a powerful flavor punch, even without the garlic used in traditional pesto. Limit servings to about 2 tablespoons per day because the pine nuts and olive oil are a little fatty. You can store this by refrigerating it in an airtight container for up to 3 days or freezing it in an ice cube tray in 1-tablespoon portions for later use.

PESTO

MAKES: ½ cup · **PREP TIME:** 5 minutes

GLUTEN-FREE
LOW-FODMAP
VEGAN

1 cup fresh basil leaves
¼ cup pine nuts
2 tablespoons olive oil
Zest of 1 lemon
½ teaspoon sea salt

In a blender or food processor, combine all the ingredients. Blend until smooth.

FLAVOR BOOST: Add ¼ cup of grated Parmesan cheese. Avoid using more than this, as the cheese can trigger acid reflux.

PER (2 TABLESPOON) SERVING: Calories: 121; Total fat: 13g; Sodium: 292mg; Carbohydrates: 2g; Fiber: 1g; Protein: 2g

This simple salad dressing blends up quickly, and it's easy to customize with flavors you like. Use a single herb or a combination of fresh herbs—some good herbs to try include cilantro, Italian parsley, oregano, chervil, thyme, rosemary, or basil. Avoid mint, which can aggravate acid reflux. This will keep in the refrigerator for up to a week.

GREEK YOGURT HERBED SALAD DRESSING

MAKES: ½ cup • **PREP TIME:** 5 minutes

GLUTEN-FREE
VEGETARIAN

¼ cup plain nonfat
  Greek yogurt
¼ cup low-fat buttermilk
¼ cup chopped fresh herb or
  herbs of your choice
1 teaspoon grated citrus zest
  (orange, lemon, or lime)
½ teaspoon sea salt

In a blender or food processor, combine all the ingredients. Blend until smooth.

———————————

INGREDIENT TIP: If you use rosemary, make sure it is cut into tiny pieces and don't include much more than about ½ teaspoon combined with other herbs, since raw fresh rosemary can impart very strong flavors.

———————————

PER (2 TABLESPOON) SERVING: Calories: 16; Total fat: <1g; Sodium: 315mg; Carbohydrates: 2g; Fiber: <1g; Protein: 2g

Dill and buttermilk are what give ranch dressing its fresh, savory, herbal flavor. This simple version uses fresh dill—feel free to add as much as you like—so if you like more herbal flavor, add more dill. You can also add up to ¼ cup of chopped fresh parsley if you like your ranch dressing with a fresh kick.

CHIVE-FREE RANCH DRESSING

MAKES: ½ cup • **PREP TIME:** 5 minutes

GLUTEN-FREE
VEGETARIAN

¼ cup buttermilk
¼ cup nonfat plain yogurt
2 tablespoons chopped fresh dill
Zest of 1 lemon
½ teaspoon sea salt

In a blender or food processor, combine all the ingredients. Blend until smooth.

SUBSTITUTION TIP: Make this dairy-free by replacing the buttermilk with an equal amount of nondairy milk and the yogurt with a nondairy plain yogurt, such as almond yogurt.

PER (2 TABLESPOON) SERVING: Calories: 13; Total fat: <1g; Sodium: 317mg; Carbohydrates: 2g; Fiber: <1g; Protein: 1g

This avocado-based salad dressing has a great orange-tarragon flavor that makes it delicious on top of greens. It's equally good as a dip, a spread for sandwiches, or even a sauce for poultry or fish. Without acid, avocado doesn't keep well and will brown relatively quickly. Preserve leftovers by storing them in a tight-sealing container with a layer of plastic wrap pressed directly down on the surface of the dressing to keep oxygen from reaching the contents.

AVOCADO-HERB SALAD DRESSING

MAKES: ½ cup • **PREP TIME:** 5 minutes

GLUTEN-FREE
VEGETARIAN

1 avocado, peeled
   and pitted
¼ cup low-fat buttermilk
¼ cup chopped
   fresh tarragon
½ teaspoon grated
   orange zest
½ teaspoon sea salt

In a blender or food processor, combine all the ingredients. Blend until smooth.

SUBSTITUTION TIP: Make this dairy-free by replacing the buttermilk with an equal amount of nondairy milk such as rice milk.

PER (2 TABLESPOON) SERVING: Calories: 83; Total fat: 7g; Sodium: 311mg; Carbohydrates: 5g; Fiber: 3g; Protein: 2g

Use this simple mayonnaise as a sandwich or burger spread or as the base for other dips and dressings. It will keep in the refrigerator for about a week, but it's best to make it in small batches and use it as you make it. You can jazz this up by adding additional flavors such as chopped fresh herbs or grated fresh ginger.

GREEK YOGURT MAYONNAISE

MAKES: ¼ cup • **PREP TIME:** 5 minutes

GLUTEN-FREE
VEGETARIAN

¼ cup nonfat plain
    Greek yogurt
1 teaspoon grated
    lemon zest
½ teaspoon sea salt

In a small bowl, combine all the ingredients. Mix well.

SUBSTITUTION TIP: You can make this low-FODMAP and dairy-free by replacing the Greek yogurt with any low-fat, nondairy plain yogurt.

PER (2 TABLESPOON) SERVING: Calories: 17; Total fat: 0g; Sodium: 593mg; Carbohydrates: 1g; Fiber: <1g; Protein: 3g

This is a tasty dip for veggies such as jicama. It's also delicious as a sandwich spread or on tacos. The ginger is soothing to acid reflux, while the cilantro is alkaline, which is also helpful for calming down GERD. It will keep in the refrigerator for up to a week, so it's best to make in smaller batches.

GINGER-CILANTRO YOGURT SPREAD/DIP

MAKES: ½ cup · **PREP TIME:** 5 minutes

GLUTEN-FREE
VEGETARIAN

¼ *cup nonfat plain yogurt*
¼ *cup finely chopped fresh cilantro*
1 tablespoon grated fresh ginger
1 teaspoon grated lime zest
½ *teaspoon sea salt*

In a small bowl, combine all the ingredients. Mix well.

FLAVOR BOOST: Add more flavor by adding up to ½ teaspoon of ground cumin, which will add a deep, smoky flavor.

PER (¼ CUP) SERVING: *Calories: 19; Total fat: <1g; Sodium: 606mg; Carbohydrates: 3g; Fiber: <1g; Protein: 2g*

Toss this simple sauce with hot pasta of any shape. This also freezes well. It's a delicious sauce to spoon over meat, poultry, or fish, so it's very versatile. Freeze in an airtight container for up to 6 months or refrigerate for about a week.

VEGETABLE PASTA SAUCE

SERVES: 4 · **PREP TIME:** 5 minutes · **COOK TIME:** 10 minutes

GLUTEN-FREE
VEGAN

2 tablespoons olive oil
1 fennel bulb, chopped
2 tablespoons fennel fronds
1 bunch asparagus, stems removed and chopped
1 tablespoon dried Italian herbs
1 cup vegetable broth, store-bought or Home-made Vegetable Broth (page 114)
½ teaspoon sea salt

1. Place a large nonstick skillet over medium-high heat and add the olive oil. Once the oil shimmers, add the fennel bulb and fronds, asparagus, and dried Italian herbs and cook, stirring occasionally, until the vegetables soften, about 4 minutes.

2. Add the broth and salt. Bring to a simmer, and then reduce the heat to medium-low. Cook until the liquid reduces by half, about 5 minutes more.

FLAVOR BOOST: Add up to ¼ cup of grated Asiago cheese to the sauce after removing the pan from the heat. Be sure you don't use any more than this, as cheese can aggravate acid reflux.

PER SERVING: Calories: 110; Total fat: 8g; Sodium: 327mg; Carbohydrates: 11g; Fiber: 5g; Protein: 4g

Pumpkin-ginger sauce is delicious on rice noodles. It's also tasty with fish or seafood or with turkey breast, so it's a versatile sauce. It freezes well, too. The alkaline pumpkin is good for calming excess acid, while ginger is a proven GERD soother.

PUMPKIN-GINGER SAUCE

SERVES: 4 · **PREP TIME:** 5 minutes · **COOK TIME:** 5 minutes

GLUTEN-FREE

VEGAN

½ *cup canned pumpkin puree (not pumpkin pie filling)*

¼ *cup vegetable broth, store-bought or Homemade Vegetable Broth (page 114)*

1 *tablespoon grated fresh ginger*

½ *teaspoon sea salt*

In a large pot, combine all the ingredients. Bring to a simmer, stirring occasionally. Cook until warmed through, about 4 minutes.

———

BATCH IT: This freezes well. Make a double or triple batch and store in ¼-cup portions in zip-top bags or airtight containers in the freezer for up to 6 months. You can also store it in 1-tablespoon portions in an ice cube tray to add to soups, meats, or sauces.

———

PER SERVING: Calories: 12; Total fat: <1g; Sodium: 293mg; Carbohydrates: 3g; Fiber: 1g; Protein: 1g

Toss this with pasta, serve it on rice, or use it as a sauce for poultry, meat, or seafood. It's a versatile sauce that brings lots of flavor to foods. Artichoke is naturally alkaline, so it's soothing for GERD. To make it lower in FODMAPs (artichokes are high-FODMAP vegetables), replace the canned artichokes with canned hearts of palm.

PUREED ARTICHOKE SAUCE

SERVES: 4 • **PREP TIME:** 5 minutes • **COOK TIME:** 5 minutes

GLUTEN-FREE
VEGETARIAN

1 (14-ounce) can artichoke bottoms, undrained
1 teaspoon grated lemon zest
½ teaspoon sea salt
¼ cup nonfat milk

1. Place the artichokes and their liquid in a large saucepan. Cook over medium-high heat until the artichokes are soft, about 5 minutes. Drain the liquid and reserve the artichokes.

2. Transfer the artichokes to a blender or food processor. Add the lemon zest, salt, and milk. Blend until smooth.

FLAVOR BOOST: Add 1 tablespoon of melted unsalted butter and ¼ cup of grated Parmesan cheese to the puree. Don't add more than this, however, as butter in large amounts can aggravate GERD.

PER SERVING: Calories: 39; Total fat: 0g; Sodium: 477mg; Carbohydrates: 8g; Fiber: 4g; Protein: 2g

This simple spread is perfect for crackers, or it's delicious as a spread on celery boats or in sandwiches. You can even use it to top baked potatoes. It's quite thick, so if you'd like a thinner consistency, add a tablespoon or two of skim milk when you blend the ingredients.

BASIL-VEGGIE SPREAD

MAKES: ½ cup • **PREP TIME:** 5 minutes

GLUTEN-FREE
VEGETARIAN

¼ cup nonfat cream cheese, at room temperature
2 tablespoons minced carrot
2 tablespoons minced fennel bulb
2 tablespoons chopped fresh basil
¼ teaspoon sea salt

In a small bowl, combine all the ingredients. Mix well.

FLAVOR BOOST: Add 2 tablespoons of minced red bell pepper.

PER (2 TABLESPOON) SERVING: Calories: 18; Total fat: 0g; Sodium: 245mg; Carbohydrates: 2g; Fiber: <1g; Protein: 2g

Tzatziki is a Greek cucumber-and-yogurt-based sauce. While cucumber can cause GERD in some people, others find its alkalinity soothing. So, proceed with caution when using this sauce unless you know cucumber isn't an acid reflux trigger for you.

TZATZIKI

MAKES: ¾ cup • **PREP TIME:** 5 minutes

GLUTEN-FREE
VEGETARIAN

½ cup nonfat plain
  Greek yogurt
¼ cup grated cucumber
1 teaspoon grated
  lemon zest
½ teaspoon sea salt

In a small bowl, combine all the ingredients. Mix well.

SUBSTITUTION TIP: If you are sensitive to cucumber, don't despair. Replace it with ¼ cup of grated zucchini or yellow summer squash.

PER (¼ CUP) SERVING: Calories: 23; Total fat: 0g; Sodium: 403mg; Carbohydrates: 2g; Fiber: <1g; Protein: 4g

With acid reflux, you may not be able to enjoy tomatoes, onions, or chile peppers, but there are other ways to make salsa. Melon makes a particularly good salsa base, and this version uses ginger and cilantro to both soothe acid reflux and pack in the flavor.

CANTALOUPE SALSA

MAKES: 2 cups • **PREP TIME:** 5 minutes

GLUTEN-FREE
VEGETARIAN

*2 cups cantaloupe
    cubes (small)*
¼ cup chopped fresh cilantro
1 tablespoon honey
*1 tablespoon grated
    fresh ginger*
1 teaspoon grated lime zest
½ teaspoon sea salt

In a small bowl, combine all the ingredients. Mix well.

─────────────

SUBSTITUTION TIP: You can make this salsa low-FODMAP by omitting the honey.

─────────────

PER (¼ CUP) SERVING: *Calories: 23; Total fat: <1g; Sodium: 150mg; Carbohydrates: 6g; Fiber: <1g; Protein: <1g*

Alkaline strawberries and soothing ginger make this a tasty toast spread that's perfect for people suffering from acid reflux. Choose strawberries that are in season for best results. You can also replace the strawberries with blackberries, raspberries, or peaches (peeled and pitted) for variations on this jam.

STRAWBERRY-GINGER FREEZER JAM

MAKES: 3 pints · **PREP TIME:** 5 minutes

GLUTEN-FREE
LOW-FODMAP
VEGETARIAN

2 cups hulled and crushed strawberries
2 tablespoons grated fresh ginger
4 cups sugar
¾ cup water
1 box Sure-Jell pectin

1. Measure exactly 2 cups of crushed strawberries into a large bowl with the grated ginger.

2. Working 1 cup at a time, stir the sugar into the strawberries, mixing well. Once all the sugar is mixed in, let rest, covered, for 10 minutes.

3. In a small saucepan, bring the water and pectin to a boil over medium-high heat, stirring constantly. Boil for 1 minute, stirring constantly; then pour into the strawberry and sugar mixture, mixing well.

4. Pour into airtight freezer containers, leaving about ½ inch at the top.

5. Cover and rest at room temperature for 24 hours.

6. Freeze for up to 1 year.

———

BATCH IT: This jam keeps very well. Make the most of strawberry season by making a double or even triple batch to enjoy for yourself and give as gifts.

————————

PER (1 TABLESPOON) SERVING: Calories: 33; Total fat: 0g; Sodium: 5mg; Carbohydrates: 9g; Fiber: <1g; Protein: 0g

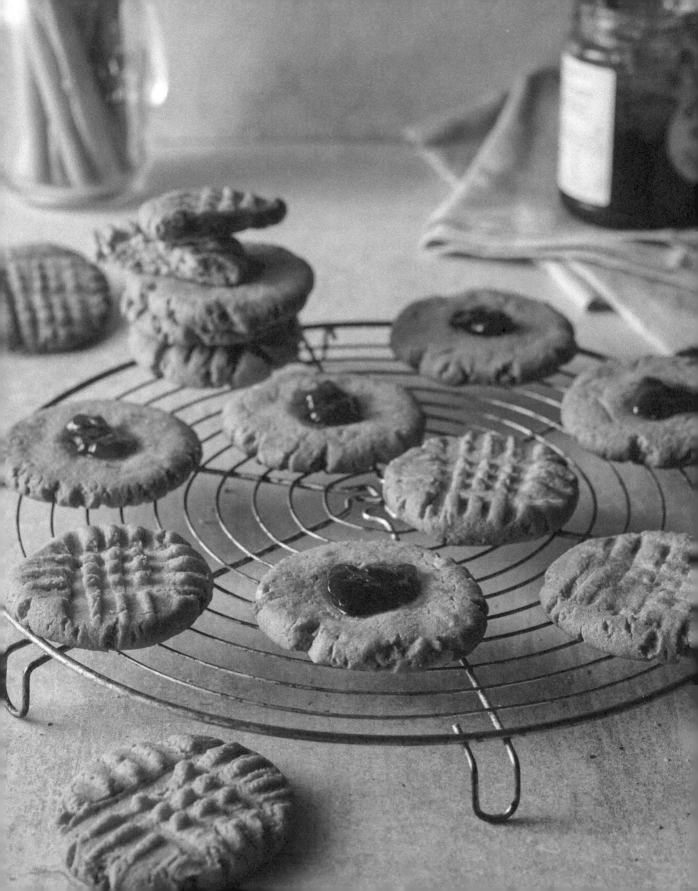

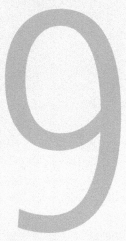

Desserts

Vanilla pudding is a delicious dessert, and it also serves as a yummy base for fresh fruit or fruit sauces. Therefore, feel free to garnish your pudding with a low-acid fruit such as blueberries, which will both add alkalinity to soothe acid reflux and gussy up the flavors of the pudding.

VANILLA PUDDING

SERVES: 6 · **PREP TIME:** 5 minutes, plus chilling time · **COOK TIME:** 10 minutes

GLUTEN-FREE
VEGETARIAN

*2¼ cups nonfat
    milk, divided*
1 teaspoon vanilla extract
Pinch sea salt
½ cup sugar
3 tablespoons cornstarch

1. In a medium saucepan, combine 2 cups of milk, the vanilla, the salt, and the sugar. Bring to a boil over medium-high heat, stirring constantly.

2. In a small bowl, whisk together the cornstarch and the remaining ¼ cup of milk.

3. Whisking constantly, pour the cornstarch mixture into the boiling milk mixture. Boil for 1 minute. Reduce the heat to low and simmer, stirring, until thick.

4. Refrigerate for 6 hours before serving.

INGREDIENT TIP: You'll be able to tell when the pudding is thick enough when you run a finger along the back of your spoon and the impression from your finger remains.

PER SERVING: Calories: 112; Total fat: <1g; Sodium: 52mg; Carbohydrates: 25g; Fiber: 0g; Protein: 3g

This is a warm, slightly spicy pudding. The ginger in it is soothing to acid reflux, and the flavor profile of orange, maple, and ginger is really delicious. This dessert is a tasty holiday treat or a good dessert anytime you're looking for a more complex flavor profile. It will keep in the refrigerator for up to a week.

MAPLE-GINGER PUDDING

SERVES: 6 · **PREP TIME:** 5 minutes, plus chilling time · **COOK TIME:** 10 minutes

GLUTEN-FREE
VEGETARIAN

2¼ cups nonfat milk, divided
1 tablespoon grated
  fresh ginger
½ cup pure maple syrup
½ teaspoon grated
  orange zest
3 tablespoons cornstarch

1. In a medium saucepan, combine 2 cups of milk, the ginger, the maple syrup, and the orange zest. Bring to a boil over medium-high heat, stirring constantly.

2. In a small bowl, whisk together the cornstarch and remaining ¼ cup of milk.

3. Whisking constantly, pour the cornstarch mixture into the boiling milk mixture. Boil for 1 minute. Reduce the heat to low and simmer, stirring, until thick.

4. Refrigerate for 6 hours before serving.

SUBSTITUTION TIP: Make this vegan and low-FODMAP by substituting a low-fat nondairy milk, such as rice milk, for the nonfat milk.

PER SERVING: *Calories: 116; Total fat: <1g; Sodium: 41mg; Carbohydrates: 26g; Fiber: 0g; Protein: 3g*

If you're a fan of the pumpkin spice trend, then you'll enjoy this pumpkin-maple custard with acid reflux–soothing ginger. To prevent a skin from forming on the custard as it chills, place plastic wrap directly on the surface of the custard. Serve topped with a dollop of fat-free vanilla yogurt.

PUMPKIN-MAPLE CUSTARD

SERVES: 6 · **PREP TIME:** 5 minutes, plus chilling time · **COOK TIME:** 10 minutes

GLUTEN-FREE
VEGETARIAN

1¾ cups nonfat milk, divided
1 tablespoon grated
   fresh ginger
½ cup pure maple syrup
½ cup pumpkin puree (not
   pumpkin pie filling)
3 tablespoons cornstarch

1. In a medium saucepan, combine 1½ cups of milk, the ginger, the maple syrup, and the pumpkin puree. Bring to a boil over medium-high heat, whisking constantly.

2. In a small bowl, whisk together the cornstarch and the remaining ¼ cup of milk.

3. Whisking constantly, pour the cornstarch mixture into the boiling milk mixture. Boil for 1 minute. Reduce the heat to low and simmer, stirring, until thick.

4. Refrigerate for 6 hours before serving.

FLAVOR BOOST: Garnish each serving with 1 tablespoon of chopped pecans to add texture and flavor. You can also add ½ teaspoon of cinnamon or pumpkin pie spice when you add the ginger.

PER SERVING: Calories: 115; Total fat: <1g; Sodium: 33mg; Carbohydrates: 26g; Fiber: 1g; Protein: 3g

Be sure to use red apples, such as Red Delicious, in this applesauce, as they are much less aggravating to acid reflux than sweet-tart apples such as Braeburn or Granny Smith. This version of applesauce is unsweetened, but if you prefer a sweeter applesauce, you can add ¼ cup of honey or pure maple syrup when you puree the apples.

GINGERED RED APPLESAUCE

SERVES: 4 • **PREP TIME:** 5 minutes • **COOK TIME:** 15 minutes

GLUTEN-FREE
VEGAN

4 red apples, peeled, cored, and chopped
¼ cup water
2 tablespoons grated fresh ginger
1 teaspoon cinnamon

1. In a large pot, bring the apples, water, ginger, and cinnamon to a boil over medium-high heat, stirring occasionally.

2. Boil, uncovered and stirring occasionally, until the apples are soft, about 10 minutes.

3. Turn off the heat and let cool.

4. Transfer the mixture to a blender or food processor and blend until smooth.

BATCH IT: This applesauce keeps well and freezes well, so feel free to double or triple the batch if you've got a large number of in-season red apples. It will keep in airtight containers in the refrigerator for up to a week or in the freezer for up to a year.

PER SERVING: Calories: 76; Total fat: <1g; Sodium: 1mg; Carbohydrates: 20g; Fiber: 4g; Protein: <1g

Freezer pops make a great dessert, and you don't need ice pop molds to make them. You can use paper cups, wooden craft sticks, and aluminum foil. Simply pour the mixture into the cups, cover them with aluminum foil, and insert the sticks through the foil. When you're ready to eat them, peel away the paper cups and foil.

GINGER-BERRY YOGURT POPS

SERVES: 4 • **PREP TIME:** 5 minutes, plus freezing time

GLUTEN-FREE
VEGETARIAN

2 cups fresh berries
2 cups plain nonfat yogurt
2 tablespoons honey
1 tablespoon grated fresh ginger

1. In a blender or food processor, combine all the ingredients. Blend until smooth.

2. Pour into molds or cups and freeze until solid, about 6 hours.

SUBSTITUTION TIP: Use any berries or combination of berries that appeal to you or are in season. You can also use other soft fruits, such as peaches or nectarines, in place of the berries.

PER SERVING: *Calories: 117; Total fat: <1g; Sodium: 81mg; Carbohydrates: 24g; Fiber: 4g; Protein: 7g*

If you're a fan of bananas Foster, then you'll likely enjoy this GERD-friendly variation on the classic. Serve it with nonfat vanilla frozen yogurt, or enjoy it by itself as a delicious dessert. Cooking the bananas adds delicious, caramelized flavors that are irresistible.

BANANAS WITH MAPLE BROWN SUGAR SAUCE

SERVES: 4 · **PREP TIME:** 5 minutes · **COOK TIME:** 10 minutes

GLUTEN-FREE

VEGAN

2 tablespoons neutral-flavored oil or coconut oil

2 bananas, peeled and split in half lengthwise, then halved crosswise

¼ cup pure maple syrup

¼ cup brown sugar

½ teaspoon cinnamon

1. Place a large nonstick skillet over medium-high heat and add the oil. Once hot, add the bananas in a single layer and cook until browned on both sides, about 5 minutes.

2. Add the maple syrup, brown sugar, and cinnamon. Cook, stirring occasionally, until the brown sugar dissolves. Serve warm.

FLAVOR BOOST: Top each serving with 1 tablespoon of chopped walnuts or macadamia nuts.

PER SERVING: *Calories: 199; Total fat: 7g; Sodium: 6mg; Carbohydrates: 39g; Fiber: 2g; Protein: 1g*

Honey and cinnamon can cool down acid reflux, and pears are alkaline. These are great warm or chilled—so if you don't want to eat them right away, store them in an airtight container in the refrigerator in the poaching liquid for up to 3 days.

HONEY-CINNAMON POACHED PEARS

SERVES: 4 · **PREP TIME:** 5 minutes · **COOK TIME:** 40 minutes

GLUTEN-FREE
VEGETARIAN

2 cups pear juice
3 tablespoons honey
2 cinnamon sticks
4 pears, peeled

1. In a large pot, bring the pear juice, honey, and cinnamon sticks to a boil over medium-high heat.

2. Add the pears and bring to a simmer. Reduce the heat to medium-low.

3. Cover and simmer until the pears are tender, about 20 minutes. Remove the pears from the liquid and set aside.

4. Bring the liquid to a boil over medium-high heat. Cook, uncovered, stirring occasionally, until the liquid is syrupy, about 10 minutes. Discard the cinnamon sticks.

5. Serve the pears warm with the syrup spooned over the top.

FLAVOR BOOST: Add 3 cardamom pods to the poaching liquid along with one 1-inch piece of ginger.

PER SERVING: Calories: 185; Total fat: <1g; Sodium: 6mg; Carbohydrates: 48g; Fiber: 5g; Protein: 1g

While pie isn't necessarily GERD-friendly, you can enjoy apple pie flavors with these yummy baked apples. Not only will the warm flavors of cinnamon and ginger soothe your acid reflux, but they are the perfect flavor to blend with apples. Your house will smell of warm spices as you cook this tasty dessert.

BAKED RED APPLES

SERVES: 4 · **PREP TIME:** 5 minutes · **COOK TIME:** 50 minutes

GLUTEN-FREE
VEGAN

4 red apples, tops cut off and cored
¼ cup brown sugar
1 teaspoon cinnamon
1 teaspoon ground ginger
4 tablespoons pure maple syrup

1. Preheat the oven to 375°F.

2. Place the apples in a 9-inch square baking pan, cut-side up.

3. In a small bowl, mix together the brown sugar, cinnamon, and ginger.

4. Spoon the mixture into the hollow core of the apples.

5. Pour 1 tablespoon of syrup over each of the apples.

6. Bake until the apples are soft, 40 to 50 minutes.

7. Serve hot.

FLAVOR BOOST: Crumble 1 graham cracker over the top of each of the baked apples and serve them with nonfat frozen vanilla yogurt.

PER SERVING: *Calories: 161; Total fat: <1g; Sodium: 6mg; Carbohydrates: 45g; Fiber: 4g; Protein: <1g*

If sundaes are your idea of the perfect dessert, then look no further than fat-free frozen vanilla yogurt topped with tasty warm blueberry sauce. You can also use other types of berries or even soft fruits such as peaches (in which case replace the sugar with brown sugar) or pears for variations on the recipe.

FROYO WITH BLUEBERRY SAUCE

SERVES: 4 · **PREP TIME:** 5 minutes · **COOK TIME:** 10 minutes

GLUTEN-FREE
VEGETARIAN

2 cups fresh blueberries
½ cup sugar
½ teaspoon grated orange zest
¼ cup water
4 scoops fat-free frozen vanilla yogurt

1. In a medium saucepan, bring the blueberries, sugar, orange zest, and water to a boil over medium-high heat, stirring often.

2. Reduce the heat to medium-low. Simmer, smashing the blueberries as you do, until the sauce thickens, about 5 minutes.

3. Cool slightly and then serve over the frozen yogurt.

───────

BATCH IT: You can make a large batch of this sauce, as it will freeze well, so it's great to make plenty when blueberries are in season. The sauce is also delicious with regular yogurt or on pancakes. Reheat it in the microwave.

───────

PER SERVING: *Calories: 226; Total fat: 0g; Sodium: 54mg; Carbohydrates: 55g; Fiber: 2g; Protein: 4g*

These super easy cookies have only four ingredients. Enjoy them as a dessert by themselves, or put a scoop of fat-free vanilla frozen yogurt in between two for an ice cream sandwich. These freeze well, so feel free to store them in a zip-top bag in the freezer for up to a year.

FLOURLESS PEANUT BUTTER COOKIES

MAKES: 15 · **PREP TIME:** 5 minutes · **COOK TIME:** 10 minutes

GLUTEN-FREE

VEGETARIAN

1 cup creamy peanut butter (or almond or cashew butter)
1 cup brown sugar
1 large egg, beaten
½ teaspoon vanilla extract

1. Preheat the oven to 350°F. Line a baking sheet with parchment paper.

2. In a medium bowl or mixer, cream together all the ingredients.

3. Drop 1-tablespoon portions of the batter on the prepared baking sheet. Use a fork to flatten the tops.

4. Bake until golden, 0 to 10 minutes.

5. Let cool for 2 minutes; then transfer to a wire rack to cool completely.

FLAVOR BOOST: Add texture by stirring in ¼ cup of chopped peanuts to the batter. You can also create a thumbprint in the middle of the cookie instead of flattening it with a fork and spoon in ½ teaspoon of jam.

PER (COOKIE) SERVING: Calories: 143; Total fat: 9g; Sodium: 88mg; Carbohydrates: 16g; Fiber: 1g; Protein: 5g

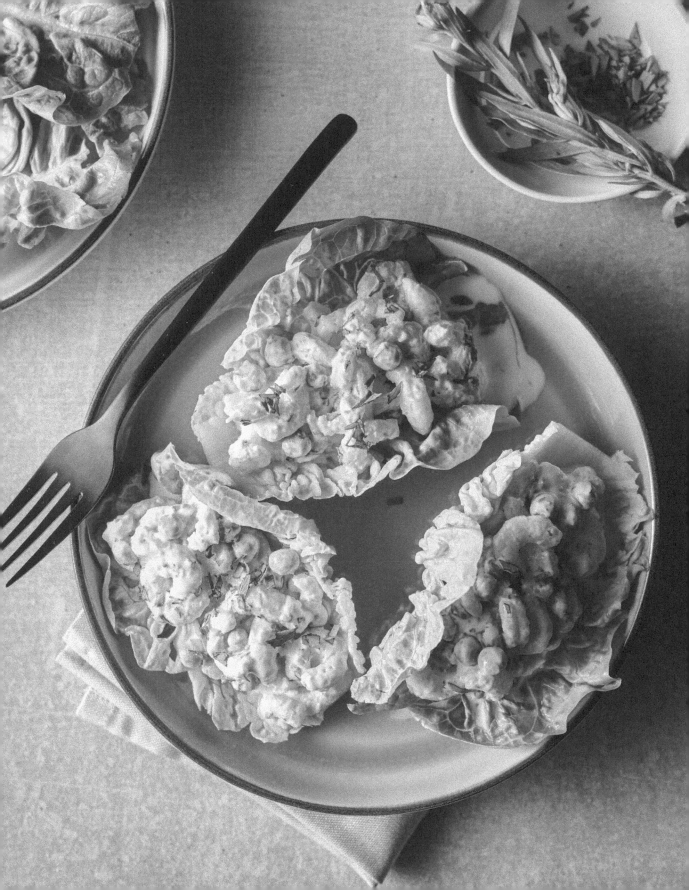

MEASUREMENT CONVERSIONS

Volume Equivalents (Liquid)

US Standard	US Standard (ounces)	Metric (approximate)
2 tablespoons	1 fl. oz.	30 mL
¼ cup	2 fl. oz.	60 mL
½ cup	4 fl. oz.	120 mL
1 cup	8 fl. oz.	240 mL
1½ cups	12 fl. oz.	355 mL
2 cups or 1 pint	16 fl. oz.	475 mL
4 cups or 1 quart	32 fl. oz.	1 L
1 gallon	128 fl. oz.	4 L

Oven Temperatures

Fahrenheit (F)	Celsius (C) (approximate)
250°F	120°C
300°F	150°C
325°F	165°C
350°F	180°C
375°F	190°C
400°F	200°C
425°F	220°C
450°F	230°C

Volume Equivalents (Dry)

US Standard	Metric (approximate)
⅛ teaspoon	0.5 mL
¼ teaspoon	1 mL
½ teaspoon	2 mL
¾ teaspoon	4 mL
1 teaspoon	5 mL
1 tablespoon	15 mL
¼ cup	59 mL
⅓ cup	79 mL
½ cup	118 mL
⅔ cup	156 mL
¾ cup	177 mL
1 cup	235 mL
2 cups or 1 pint	475 mL
3 cups	700 mL
4 cups or 1 quart	1 L

Weight Equivalents

US Standard	Metric (approximate)
½ ounce	15 g
1 ounce	30 g
2 ounces	60 g
4 ounces	115 g
8 ounces	225 g
12 ounces	340 g
16 ounces or 1 pound	455 g

REFERENCES

American College of Gastroenterology. "Acid Reflux." gi.org/topics/acid-reflux.

de Bortoli, Nicola, Giada Guidi, Katia Nardi, Alessandra Stella, Salvatore Tolone, Marzio Frazzoni, Leonardo Frazzoni, Lorenzo Fuccio, Massimo Bellini, Vincenzo Savarino, Santino Marchi, and Edoardo V. Savarino. "Low-FODMAP Diet Resulted Effective in Relieving Esophageal and Intestinal Symptoms in Patients with Pathophysiological Characteristics of Functional Heartburn and a Prospective, Interventional Study." *Gastroenterology* 152, no. 5 (2017): S751.

Eherer, A. J., F. Netolitzky, C. Högenauer, G. Puschnig, T. A. Hinterleitner, S. Scheidl, W. Kraxner, G. J. Krejs, and K. M. Hoffmann. "Positive Effect of Abdominal Breathing Exercise on Gastroesophageal Reflux Disease: A Randomized, Controlled Study." *American Journal of Gastroenterology* 107, no. 3 (2012): 372–78.

El-Serag, H. B., J. A. Satia, and L. Rabeneck. "Dietary Intake and the Risk of Gastro-Oesophageal Reflux Disease: A Cross Sectional Study in Volunteers." *Gut* 54, no. 1 (2005): 11–17.

Fujiwara, Y., A. Machida, Y. Watanabe, M. Shiba, K. Tominaga, T. Watanabe, N. Oshitani, K. Higuchi, and T. Arakawa. "Association between Dinner-to-Bed Time and Gastro-Esophageal Reflux Disease." *American Journal of Gastroenterology* 100, no. 12 (2005): 2633–36.

Hosseini, M., R. Salari, M. Akbari Rad, M. Salehi, B. Birjandi, and M. Salari. "Comparing the Effect of Psyllium Seed on Gastroesophageal Reflux Disease with Oral Omeprazole in Patients with Functional Constipation." *Journal of Evidence-Based Integrative Medicine* 23 (2018). https://doi.org/10.1177/2515690X18763294.

Jarosz, M., and A. Taraszewska. "Risk Factors for Gastroesophageal Reflux Disease: The Role of Diet." *Przegląd Gastroenterologiczny* 9, no. 5 (2014): 297–301.

Kandil, Tharwat S., Amany A. Mousa, Ahmed A. El-Gendy, and Amr M. Abbas. "The Potential Therapeutic Effect of Melatonin in Gastro-Esophageal Reflux Disease." *BMC Gastroenterology* 10, no. 7 (2010): 1–9.

Kristianslund, C. H., J. G. Hatlebakk, T. Hausken, M. H. Morken, and G. E. Kahrs. "PP083-SUN: Effect of FODMAP-Restricted Diet on Gastroesophageal Reflux Disease." *Clinical Nutrition* 33 (2014): S50.

Maradey-Romero, Carla, Hemangi Kale, and Ronnie Fass. "Nonmedical Therapeutic Strategies for Nonerosive Reflux Disease." *Journal of Clinical Gastroenterology* 48, no. 7 (2014): 584–89.

Morozov, S., V. Isakov, and M. Konovalova. "Fiber-Enriched Diet Helps to Control Symptoms and Improves Esophageal Motility in Patients with Non-Erosive Gastroesophageal Reflux Disease." *World Journal of Gastroenterology* 24, no. 21 (2018): 2291–99.

Nocon, M., J. Labenz, and S. N. Willich. "Lifestyle Factors and Symptoms of Gastro-Oesophageal Reflux—a Population-Based Study." *Alimentary Pharmacology & Therapeutics* 23, no. 1 (2006): 169–74.

Piesman, M., I. Hwang, C. Maydonovitch, and R. K. Wong. "Nocturnal Reflux Episodes Following the Administration of a Standardized Meal. Does Timing Matter?" *American Journal of Gastroenterology* 102 (2007): 2128–34.

Shaheen, Nicholas J. "Highlights from the New ACG Guidelines for the Diagnosis and Management of GERD." *Gastroenterology & Hepatology* 9, no. 6 (2013): 377–79.

Xu, L., X. Zhang, J. Lu, J. X. Dai, R. Q. Lin, F. X. Tian, B. Liang, et al. "The Effects of Dinner-to-Bed Time and Post-Dinner Walk on Gastric Cancer across Different Age Groups: A Multicenter Case-Control Study in Southeast China." *Medicine* (Baltimore) 95, no. 16 (2016): e3397.

Yamasaki, T., C. Hemond, M. Eisa, S. Ganocy, and R. Fass. "The Changing Epidemiology of Gastroesophageal Reflux Disease: Are Patients Getting Younger?" *Journal of Neurogastroenterology and Motility* 24, no. 14 (2018): 559–69.

Yang, J. H., H. S. Kang, S. Y. Lee, J. H. Kim, I. K. Sung, H. S. Park, C. S. Shim, and C. J. Jin. "Recurrence of Gastroesophageal Reflux Disease Correlated with a Short Dinner-to-Bedtime Interval." *Journal of Gastroenterology and Hepatology* 29, no. 4 (2014): 730–35.

Zalvan, Craig H., Shirley Hu, Barbara Greenberg, and Jan Geliebter. "A Comparison of Alkaline Water and Mediterranean Diet Vs. Proton Pump Inhibition for Treatment of Laryngopharyngeal Reflux." *JAMA Otolaryngology–Head & Neck Surgery* 143, no. 10 (2017): 1023–29.

Zhang, C. X., Y. M. Qin, and B. R. Guo. "Clinical Study on the Treatment of Gastroesophageal Reflux by Acupuncture." *Chinese Journal of Integrative Medicine* 16, no. 4 (2010): 298–303.

INDEX

Page locators in **bold** indicate picture

ACKNOWLEDGMENTS

This particular book happens to be my fifth and perhaps the one I resonate with the most because I personally appreciate the quality-of-life improvements that come with the improved management of GERD and other gastrointestinal conditions.

With that being said, I want to thank those of you who have purchased this book and put some faith in what I have to say regarding this condition.

I did my very best to assess the available scientific evidence surrounding the dietary management of GERD, and I sincerely hope that the guidance within complements your current healthcare protocol and serves to improve your daily life and overall health going forward.

All the best,
Andy De Santis, RD, MPH

ABOUT THE AUTHOR

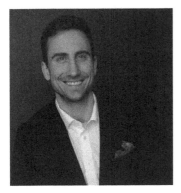

Andy De Santis, RD, MPH, is a registered dietitian, speaker, and five-time author from Toronto, Canada. He operates a private dietetics practice focused on customized nutrition solutions for people dealing with a wide variety of issues and prides himself on providing exceptional care to his clients. Andy has been featured in local newspapers and magazines and on television. He is never afraid to provide his views on topics of importance. When he isn't helping people in a one-on-one setting, Andy loves creating hard-hitting content with a lighthearted twist, which he shares through his personal blog, AndyTheRD.com, and various social media accounts, including Instagram (@AndyTheRD).

Printed in the USA
CPSIA information can be obtained
at www.ICGtesting.com
LVHW072325101123
763346LV00002B/19